Clinical Trials

*What Patients and Healthy Volunteers
Need to Know*

Clinical Trials

What Patients and Healthy Volunteers Need to Know

LORNA SPEID, PhD, BPharm, MRPharmS

OXFORD
UNIVERSITY PRESS
2010

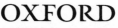

OXFORD
UNIVERSITY PRESS

Oxford University Press, Inc., publishes works that further
Oxford University's objective of excellence
in research, scholarship, and education.

Oxford New York
Auckland   Cape Town   Dar es Salaam   Hong Kong   Karachi
Kuala Lumpur   Madrid   Melbourne   Mexico City   Nairobi
New Delhi   Shanghai   Taipei   Toronto

With offices in
Argentina   Austria   Brazil   Chile   Czech Republic   France   Greece
Guatemala   Hungary   Italy   Japan   Poland   Portugal   Singapore
South Korea   Switzerland   Thailand   Turkey   Ukraine   Vietnam

Copyright © 2010 by Oxford University Press, Inc.

Published by Oxford University Press, Inc.
198 Madison Avenue, New York, New York 10016
www.oup.com

Oxford is a registered trademark of Oxford University Press, Inc.

Library of Congress Cataloging-in-Publication Data

Speid, Lorna.
   Clinical trials: what patients and healthy volunteers need to know / by
Lorna Speid.
      p. cm.
   ISBN 978-0-19-973416-0
   1.   Clinical trials—Popular works.   I. Title.
   R853.C55S625 2010
   615.5072'4—dc22

                                                            2010009154

9 8 7 6 5 4 3 2 1
Printed in the United States of America
on acid-free paper

To my mother, Icilda Valieri DeGouttes Speid,
a continuing inspiration

Foreword

A Google search using the keyword "clinical trial" yields 29,400,000 hits (in 0.19 seconds). This daunting amount of information makes it nearly impossible for an individual interested in participating in a clinical trial to negotiate the morass of medical terms, complex acronyms, and difficult-to-understand regulatory requirements, or to foster and encourage participation in clinical research. This is perhaps just one of many reasons why participation in clinical research has not been a national priority; as a consequence, for example, less than 5% of adult cancer patients are currently enrolled in clinical trials (Keller et al., 2007).

Clinical trial accrual rates for oncology trials are therefore currently inadequate, resulting in delays in scientific progress against cancer as well as other diseases. In a recent study published in the *Journal of Clinical Oncology*, clinical trials were never even mentioned in 43% of interactions between physicians and their cancer patients (Albrecht et al., 2008). Moreover, the pool of willing patients is further reduced by the reluctance of some physicians to engage in participation in clinical research (Comis, Miller, Aldigé, Krebs, & Stoval, 2003).

Putting these statistics into context, it is notable that participation in clinical trials among pediatric cancer patients exceeds 90% nationally. Clearly this high fraction of participation in clinical research has been beneficial inasmuch as childhood leukemia used to be a devastating killer disease in pediatric populations prior to the advent of suitable treatment modalities aimed at eradicating leukemia. However, childhood leukemia now boasts a greater than 95% cure rate. The connection between patient participation in clinical research and dramatic improvements in the cure rate for this deadly disease is no coincidence. Therefore, it behooves us as a society to take greater interest in design, conduct, and participation in clinical research in order to accelerate the pace of medical discoveries and eradication or control of deadly diseases.

In her book *Clinical Trials: What Patients and Healthy Volunteers Need to Know*, Dr. Lorna Speid has produced an authoritative and complete resource that, despite the complexities of clinical research, is easy to read and understand. The book is rich in illustrations, figures, links to relevant Web sites, and definitions of complex medical terminology. Thus, in my opinion her book can be viewed as "one-stop shopping" for patients interested in participation in clinical trials, and I would argue that this book should be a resource available on coffee tables in doctors' office waiting rooms worldwide. Given the busy and complex schedules of practicing clinicians, it is often the patient who dictates discussion about participation in clinical research rather than the physician; therefore, if the patient is not knowledgeable or aware of the possibilities of clinical trials, he or she would necessarily not be empowered to bring this up in conversations with personal physicians in order to explore possible experimental options for treatment of difficult diseases.

I have had the pleasure of working firsthand with the author several years ago in the planning, design, and conduct of a first-in-man Phase

I clinical trial of an experimental anticancer agent, and as a result of our collaboration, I can assure that Dr. Speid is an authority on the subject of clinical research and current regulatory requirements for design and conduct of clinical trials.

In summary, I consider *Clinical Trials: What Patients and Healthy Volunteers Need to Know* a must read for patients, families, and even medical professionals who are contemplating involvement in clinical research. Increasing knowledge and awareness of availability of clinical trials empowers patients and their families to take advantage of new and cutting-edge medical research. This research will foster and encourage the pace of discovery in medical research, which historically has sometimes proceeded at a frustratingly slow pace. Another value added for participation in clinical research is the reassurance that the treatment will involve at least "standard of care" medical practice with considerable regulatory oversight of the interactions between physicians and patients. And it guarantees input from an ethics committee as well as written and verbal communication from a physician and researchers to the patient regarding the expectations as well as potential pitfalls for participation in clinical trials. Only such open and honest communication between the medical research community and patients can overcome historical and cultural barriers that have confounded active participation in clinical trials for the majority of eligible patients in the United States. It is therefore my distinct pleasure to recommend this work as a solution to the challenge of patient participation in clinical research.

Mark D. Pegram, M.D.
Sylvester Professor of Medicine
Division of Hematology/Oncology
Director, Clinical and Translational Research
Braman Family Breast Cancer Research Institute
University of Miami Sylvester Comprehensive Cancer Center
University of Miami Miller School of Medicine

References

Albrecht, T. L., Eggly, S. S., Gleason, M. E. J., Harper, F. W. K., Foster, T. S., Peterson, A. M., et al. (2008). Influence of clinical communication on patients' decision making on participation in clinical trials. *Journal of Clinical Oncology, 26*(16), 2666–2673.

Comis, R. L., Miller, J. D., Aldigé, C. R., Krebs, L., & Stoval, E. (2003). Public attitudes toward participation in cancer clinical trials. *Journal of Clinical Oncology, 21*(5), 830–835.

Keller, J. K., Bowman, J., Lee, J. A., Frisby, K. A., Mathiason, M. A., Meyer, C. M., et al. (2007). Poor access to clinical trials among newly diagnosed adult cancer patients in the community—1999–2004. *Community Oncology, 4*(11), 695–700.

Acknowledgments

Many people are responsible for making this book a reality. I must of course thank the many clinical trial patients and their relatives with whom I have been involved over the years. They were truly my inspiration. I am also grateful to Oxford University Press and, in particular, Joan Bossert for believing in this book. She immediately saw its value and championed it through the process of review. In addition, Aaron van Dorn and Abby Gross were instrumental in the day-to-day editing and perfecting of the manuscript.

I am honored that Dr. Mark Pegram has written the Foreword. I have watched him in action with patients as well as behind the scenes as we planned and prepared for clinical trials. He is an exceptional physician, and I admire what he does for patients and their families.

I am thankful for the advice of Jeff Herman, a professional agent who believed in the project and guided me through the process of seeking a publisher. Dr. Suzanne Kennedy pointed me in the direction of university publishers, which eventually led me to Oxford University Press. Thank you, Suzanne.

Barrington Downie reviewed an earlier version of the manuscript and proved to be a valuable sounding board as the project was taking shape. Dr. Lynne Eddy is a fellow life sciences consultant and spent time reviewing critical chapters and providing thorough, invaluable input. My dear friend Susan Cornelius had firsthand experience of a childhood cancer situation and was invaluable as I developed the pediatric chapter. Dr. Anthony Fox, pharmaceutical physician and expert in drug development, provided excellent input as a reviewer. Dr. Sean Sullivan, expert in gene therapy, provided helpful feedback on the gene therapy chapter. Dr. Michael P. Caligiuri, professor in residence and director of the Human Research Protections Program at the University of California San Diego, engaged me in very helpful discussions on the chapters involving the role of the institutional review board.

Finally, I appreciate the time taken by the following physician reviewers to review the final manuscript and write reviews:

Gioi N. Smith-Nguyen, MD, FACOG., Diplomate American Board of Obstetrics & Gynecology, Director and Principal Investigator, Grossmont Center for Clinical Research, La Mesa, California.

David A. Williams, MD, Chief of the Division of Hematology/ Oncology, Director of Translational Research for Children's Hospital Boston and Leland Fikes Professor of Pediatrics, Harvard Medical School.

David A. Merrill, MD, PhD, Investigator, Division of Geriatric Psychiatry, Memory & Aging Research Center, Semel Institute for Neuroscience & Human Behaviour David Geffen School of Medicine at University of California, Los Angeles.

Contents

CONTENTS

Clinical Trials

*What Patients and Healthy Volunteers
Need to Know*

Why I Wrote This Book

I had moved to the United States from Europe a few months before to work for a small biotechnology company in a beautiful place called The Woodlands, in Texas. As a project leader, it was my job to lead the effort to develop a gene therapy for the treatment of head and neck cancers. I was responsible for preparing the documentation that would be submitted to the Food and Drug Administration, as well as the hospital sites where we intended to conduct clinical trials. To update my knowledge of the cutting edge treatments available for the treatment of head and neck cancer, I had arranged to spend two days shadowing physicians at a prominent Houston institution considered amongst the pioneers for the treatment of head and neck cancer. So, here I was, sitting in the common area where the physicians were busy dictating their notes following meetings with patients, some of them terminally ill. When I wasn't sitting in this room, I was shadowing the chief physician or one of the physicians on a fellowship at the hospital.

The Chief physician was a jovial man, worshipped by his patients. He clearly had a knack for putting patients at ease, and for making them believe that they would be alright despite their cancer diagnoses. He painstakingly took his time with each patient, and explained the proposed treatment to them, or reviewed the results of any treatments already received. I observed as he compassionately found ways around their insurance challenges to ensure that their treatment could proceed without the hindrance of unnecessary insurance bureaucracy. Many of these patients would be placed on clinical trials run by the institution or pharmaceutical companies.

As I shadowed the physicians I began to ponder how difficult it must be to take in a diagnosis of cancer, as well as information being presented about the clinical trials which many of the patients were being enrolled into. It seemed as though much of the information must go in one ear and out of the other.

I have played an active role in the design, setup, and conduct of clinical trials on behalf of the pharmaceutical industry. It is a complicated process, even for the professionals working within it. Inundated by jargon and scientific terminology that are difficult to understand, I can imagine most people feel intimidated by the process, especially if they are also dealing with a chronic or serious illness. One of the reasons that I wrote this book was to empower the patients and healthy volunteers, otherwise known as research subjects, who participate in clinical trials. Research subjects must take responsibility for their safety during participation in clinical trials. This must be done in partnership with other professionals involved with clinical trial oversight. Knowledge empowers. In this case, knowledge will empower research subjects to critically evaluate safety information presented to them, and to make decisions about their safety within a clinical trial. Knowledge will also enable you as the research subject to realistically estimate the potential for benefit from participating in a specific clinical trial.

Before a research subject takes part in a clinical trial, they are required to give their informed consent. Informed consent implies that the person giving consent understands what they are consenting to. All too often, when research subjects are involved in medical incidents that result in injuries during clinical trials, they or their representatives state that they were not told about the risks involved in participating in the clinical trial, and that had they understood the risks, they would not have participated. So often, information presented in informed consent documents is difficult to understand by those for whom they were written. There is little available background information on the process of informed consent and related matters for research subjects. A search of the internet for clinical trial information will produce many "hits." Unfortunately, much of the information found will be biased, difficult to sift through, and generally unhelpful. I wrote this book to provide a systematic and easy to follow explanation of the clinical trial process. Not only does the book explain the process, but it also provides a useful guide on where to look for additional information on the internet (Chapter 14). While research subjects who are competent mentally and emotionally must take the responsibility for their own participation in a clinical trial, caregivers must take this responsibility on behalf of those who are not competent to do so, including children (Chapters 10, 11 and 13).

You may be reading this book because you are considering taking part in a clinical trial, or you may already be involved in a trial. Another possibility is that someone whom you care about is currently taking part in a clinical trial or is considering taking part in a clinical trial. Either way you are likely to have many questions that you would like answered. The medical professionals involved in the trial process can only answer the questions that you ask. If you don't know which questions you should ask, or if you feel too intimidated to ask questions, you will be doing yourself a great disservice. I wrote this book to help you identify some of the questions you should ask before and after signing the informed consent document. A list of suggested questions is provided within the chapters when appropriate. These questions will help you to hold a meaningful conversation with the physician overseeing the clinical trial.

Although the book is written at a level that should be easy to read, there will undoubtedly be scientific concepts and principles that are difficult to understand. A glossary is provided at the end of the book so that you can look up any terms that you have not come across before. When the term "drug" is used in this book, it is used as a catchall. You should assume that the principles being discussed will apply to new medicines, devices, diagnostics, gene therapy, as well as experimental therapies and approaches to treating diseases.

The Chief of Head and Neck Cancer was now introducing me to the patient in front of us and informing her that I worked for a pharmaceutical company that was conducting research to find a cure for head and neck cancer. The patient nodded gratefully to me. Many years would pass before I would finally put pen to paper and begin the process of writing the book that you are now reading. I would like to think that that patient might one day read it.

★★★

Some readers may not wish to read this book from cover to cover. Other readers may choose to read the sections that are most needed for their particular situation. I encourage you to keep this book with you for your visits during the clinical trial. Use it as a reference book. During your clinical trial visits, check the Glossary when an investigator uses a term that you have not heard before.

Understanding Clinical Trials

2

Several years ago, I visited a facility in the United Kingdom that conducted Phase 1 clinical trials in healthy volunteers. The facility was located in a busy part of London. I was given a tour of a nice modern facility that had areas where the healthy volunteers could congregate and watch television or play cards and board games. The study staff consisted of several nurses, a coordinator, and a physician. Study sponsors would contract with this facility to test their drugs in research subjects and to provide the results. The healthy volunteers were examined according to the clinical protocol at specified intervals, and the results were written down carefully on special forms. Between the drug administration and examinations the healthy volunteers were free to lie down on the beds organized in dormitory style or to go about their day-to-day activities within the dormitory setting or in the common areas. Many of the healthy volunteers that were there on the day of my visit appeared to be university students. This particular facility was situated close to a general hospital and could therefore access emergency medical care if there were any unexpected reactions.

What Are Clinical Trials?

A clinical trial is a study that is carried out on human beings to determine how safe a drug is and, if the study is designed adequately, how well the drug works. Clinical trials are carried out in two types of research subjects. The first are research subjects who do not have the disease being studied; these are known as healthy volunteers. The second are research subjects who have the disease being studied, or patients.

Studies conducted in healthy volunteers are known as Phase 1 studies. They are sometimes referred to as "first-in-man studies" if the drug has not been studied previously in humans. The goal of these studies is to determine the pharmacological and pharmacokinetic effects of the drug, often at very low doses.

The goal of a clinical trial that is conducted in patients is to conduct a controlled study of the effectiveness and safety of a drug. This is accomplished by studying a representative group of research subjects. The results of the clinical trial can then be extrapolated to the wider affected patient population. For instance, patients with colorectal cancer will be studied in clinical trials to determine if the drug that is being developed can be used to treat patients with colorectal cancer. The number of patients that must be studied in a clinical trial in order to represent the wider population is defined by statistical concepts, which will not be considered in detail in this book.

Why Do We Need Clinical Trials?

Tests in laboratories and on animals can only suggest a drug's potential to treat a disease or condition effectively. Tests on animals are not sufficient to confirm if the drug works because animals are not exact replicas of human beings. An effect that is observed in animals may not be seen in humans because of species differences. Studies must therefore be carried out in humans even after extensive studies have been carried out in animals. The animal studies help to guide the doses to be used in clinical trials and can provide insight into how the clinical trials should be designed.

Examples of Different Types of Clinical Trials

There are different types of clinical trials as shown below, although this list is not exhaustive:

- Clinical trials are carried out on new drugs that have not previously been commercialized for use in patients.
- Clinical trials are conducted to find new uses for old medicines. For instance, aspirin is used to prevent heart attacks, although it was initially developed for use as a painkiller. Clinical trials helped to establish that aspirin could be used in the treatment and prevention of cardiovascular disease, myocardial infarction, and stroke.
- Combinations of marketed medicines can sometimes be more effective than the individual medicines on their own. New combinations of established medicines may be tested in clinical trials. Many cancer treatments are used in combination. Tuberculosis (TB) and human immunodeficiency virus (HIV) treatments are also always used in combination.
- Medical devices are tested in clinical trials before they are sold. An example of a medical device is an electrocardiographic (ECG) machine, which is used to monitor the heart.
- Diagnostic tests are used to identify diseases that patients are suffering from. Before a new diagnostic procedure is routinely used, it will be

studied in clinical trials. Some examples of diagnostic tests are those that test the level of sugar in the blood or in the urine. As new ways to screen patients become available, clinical trials are often used to determine the accuracy and safety of these techniques and whether they perform consistently from one patient to another. For example, a magnetic resonance imaging (MRI) machine was studied in clinical trials before it could be used in clinical practice.

Who Conducts and Sponsors Clinical Trials and in What Settings?

Clinical trials may be sponsored by physicians, private research institutions, government research institutions such as the National Institutes of Health (NIH), university hospitals, and the pharmaceutical industry, just to name a few types of organizations. These organizations are known as "sponsors."

Clinical trial sponsors may have different motivations and goals for sponsoring clinical trials. For instance, a pharmaceutical industry sponsor will have the main motivation of ultimately commercializing the drug that is being studied. A physician or a group of physicians conducting a clinical trial in their offices may have the goal of publishing a paper on a new chemical entity or a commercialized drug. University hospitals may conduct clinical trials to develop a better understanding of how to use currently available treatments for diseases in which they specialize. For instance, many of the currently used combination treatments for the treatment of HIV and cancer are developed and tested by hospital institutions in their own clinical trials. The physicians that take part in these clinical trials may publish their findings, with the goal of influencing clinical practice. These physicians may be recognized for their expertise and sought after by their peers. Government agencies may also conduct specialized clinical trials.

For example, the Department of Veterans Affairs in the United States might run studies to test vaccines against germs that soldiers may be exposed to during war time. In short, the motivations and purposes of clinical research will be different in different settings. These factors need to be borne in mind as one considers the clinical trial, where it is being conducted, and who is sponsoring it.

Different types of organizations may be involved in the day-to-day conduct and oversight of clinical trials. Sponsors may hire clinical research organizations (CROs) to conduct all or part of the clinical trial on their behalf. For instance, a sponsor may hire a CRO to conduct a portion of a multinational clinical trial in a part of the world where the sponsor does not have offices and staff. Although the CRO will conduct all or parts of the clinical trial, the sponsor is still responsible for how the study is conducted and for ensuring that the necessary regulations and guidelines are complied with in each territory in which the clinical trial is conducted. It may not be evident when a CRO is involved with the conduct of the clinical trial because the named organization will likely be the study sponsor rather than the CRO that is working for the sponsor.

In the United States, general clinical research centers (GCRCs) form a national network and provide support to investigators to assure that clinical research is conducted to high standards. The term *GCRC* may be used to describe the facility within which the clinical trial will be conducted. The investigators that conduct their studies within the GCRCs receive financial support from the NIH or other federal agencies. It is also permissible for healthy volunteers or patients to stay overnight within a GCRC for studies involving some hospitalization. General clinical research centers are also involved in studies requiring outpatient care, or some in-hospital and outpatient care.

Another term used in clinical trial circles is *site management organization* (SMO). These organizations manage the investigative sites and help to ensure that each site is able to conduct the clinical trial to the appropriate standards.

Tests in animals and in vitro can only give so much information about a drug. Studies must be carried out in humans in order to determine the safety and efficacy of the drug. These studies are known as clinical trials. In the next chapter we will consider how clinical trials are regulated.

Oversight of Clinical Trials

3

There is an old joke that goes something like "I am from the government, and I am here to help you!" Sadly, many people associate their national government with bureaucracy and taxes instead of protection. In the area of oversight of clinical trials, a national regulatory or health authority that is a part of the government plays a critical role in keeping research subjects safe and in ensuring that appropriate standards are followed by sponsors. In this case, a well-functioning regulatory authority really is here to help. Regulatory authorities share oversight with committees that oversee the ethics, safety, and scientific rigor of clinical research known as ethics committees. Ethics committees are known as institutional review boards (IRBs) in the United States.

Who Regulates the Conduct of Clinical Trials?

Regulatory authorities exist to monitor the safety and effectiveness of medicines and to ensure that any claims that companies make for their products are valid. Regulatory authorities issue guidelines on the types of clinical trials to be carried out for different types of disease. For instance, the Food and Drug Administration is the regulatory authority that regulates the development of new drugs in the United States. Examples of other regulatory authorities around the world are the Medicines and Healthcare Products Regulatory Agency (United Kingdom), European Medicines Agency (European Union), Ministry of Health and Welfare (Japan), Health Canada (Canada), Therapeutic Goods Administration (Australia), Public Health Institute (Russia), Swiss Agency for Therapeutic Products (Switzerland), and Ministry of Health of the People's Republic of China (China). Space prevents me from listing every regulatory authority, but suffice it to say that the regulation of medicines is a priority for these regulatory authorities.

Sponsors of clinical trials must apply to regulatory authorities for authorization to conduct clinical trials. In the United States this authorization is known as an investigational new drug (IND). In other countries, it is known as a clinical trial application or authorization (CTA). In the United States, physicians may also conduct clinical trials under physician-initiated IND applications.

Toxicology studies must be carried out (in animals) before a drug can be tested in humans. The toxicology guidelines varied from country to country until the early 1990s. Initiatives by the major regulatory authorities under the auspices of the International Conference on Harmonization (ICH) have reduced the number of differences in toxicology and other areas of drug development between countries, although there are still some differences that sponsors have to work through in order to register their drugs in as many countries as possible.

After all clinical trials have been carried out on a drug in accordance with the regulatory guidelines and the information has been gathered during the animal studies, clinical trials must be summarized in detailed reports that describe how the studies were carried out and how the results were obtained. These reports are then submitted to regulatory

14

authorities to seek approval to market the drug. This process is repeated in as many different countries as possible. It is through registration in as many countries as possible that money spent on research and development is recuperated (see Chapter 8). In addition to regulating the testing of new drugs and medical treatments, regulatory authorities provide advice and input to researchers to help them to design high-quality drug development programs (see Chapter 8).

Ethics Committees

In addition to regulatory authorities, ethics committees (ECs) oversee the progress of clinical trials. They monitor the safety, rights, and welfare of participants. The people that sit on the ECs may be from diverse backgrounds. They are typically a mix of scientists, non scientists, people trained in ethics, people with legal or clergy backgrounds, and lay members of the community. The method used to select these individuals may be determined by the hospital or clinical facility in which the research is conducted. In the United States, the IRB consists of at least five individuals and may have additional consultants to assist with more complex drugs if the IRB needs expert input to assure an adequate review.

The job of the EC is to evaluate the clinical research and to point out ethical and safety issues to the investigator that must be addressed before the clinical research may start. In each individual country, the operation and functioning of ECs may be defined in regulations and laws. For example, in the European Union (EU), the functioning and operation of ECs is defined in Directive 2001/20/EC. The Directive sets strict time limits within which the review of a clinical protocol must be completed. Each individual country within the European Union has written the requirements of the Directive into the national law. Single investigative sites will usually have an EC associated with it, or upon which it can call for the review of protocols. For multinational clinical trials conducted in different countries within the EU, each individual country has a system to ensure that a single opinion will be provided for the clinical protocol conducted in the country. In the United States, the role and function of the IRB is described in detail in 21 Code of Federal Regulations 56, which is available on the Internet.

Different countries have different systems for how submissions should be made to the ECs in the country and within what time-frames. For instance, in the United States, when many investigative sites will be involved in a clinical trial, the sponsor can arrange for a centralized IRB to conduct the review of the protocol and associated documentation. The centralized IRB will coordinate with the IRBs at each investigative site to decide how the responsibilities for oversight of the clinical trial will be shared.

Ethics committees meet on a regular basis. Submissions must be made in time for consideration at the scheduled meetings. Procedurally, the EC may meet formally so that its members can review the data package provided for review by the investigator. Packages of documents related to the clinical trial will usually be sent to members for review several days to several weeks before the actual meeting takes place. The sponsor will submit the protocol, investigator's brochure, informed consent document, and supporting documentation to the EC to seek permission to conduct the clinical trial. If there are no objections, a written approval will be given for the study to proceed. The EC may request changes to the informed consent document or the protocol before granting approval for the study to proceed, or it may determine that the study is unsafe or unethical and should not proceed. The study cannot proceed until the approval is obtained from the EC *and* the regulatory authority. A regulatory authority can disallow an EC-approved clinical trial, but the regulatory authority cannot allow an EC-disapproved trial to proceed.

If a provisional approval is granted contingent upon changes to the clinical protocol or to the informed consent document, the start of the study may be delayed until the complete IRB or EC can meet again. At times, if the change requested to the clinical protocol or the informed consent document was minor, the IRB or EC chairperson may be able to grant the final approval without the need for the committee to meet again in full.

Although physicians and investigators may sit on an EC, members of an EC should have no vested interest in the outcome of the deliberations that take place at meetings. Therefore, principal investigators (PIs) or investigators who normally sit on an EC cannot deliberate or vote on protocols that they are themselves involved with, or if they have a conflict of interest with the project or the PI conducting the study.

After the study has been approved and may begin, the PI will need to provide the EC with regular updates and reports on any adverse events. During the clinical trial, the EC will assess the way that the clinical trial is carried out to make sure that the required standards continue to be followed on an ongoing basis. During the clinical trial, ECs will seek to minimize the risks to which research subjects are exposed, and to balance these against the potential for benefit. The EC can stop the study if it is not being carried out according to the clinical protocol, or if the risks of the study are determined to be too great (see Chapter 5).

The ECs must ensure that the research subjects are selected according to the clinical protocol, and that their safety is being adequately monitored. The EC must also ensure that subjects are not enrolled in clinical trials before they have given their informed consent, and that all changes in the protocol proposed by investigators or sponsors are approved by the EC before they are implemented. The EC will seek to ensure that the latest informed consent document reflects the latest clinical protocol.

During the clinical trial, the PI will send correspondence to the EC and respond to any questions or comments about the ongoing clinical trial in writing. The unexpected serious adverse events that are considered related to the drug must be reported by the investigator to the EC in an expedited fashion. These will be sent to the EC in writing. The PI may be asked to meet with the EC in person to provide a status update on the clinical trial that was previously approved.

A single clinical trial can be carried out at many different investigative sites in a single country or in many different countries. A sponsor must assign an experienced project manager to manage the process of submission to the IRBs and ECs in each individual country in which the protocol is to be conducted. For instance, a sponsor may wish to work with several investigators in the United States and several investigators in countries across the globe. Each protocol submission will generate its own correspondence. The submission process may vary from country to country. As the EC considers the protocol, questions may be sent back to the sponsor for response. Each set of questions will need to be responded to within a reasonable timeframe to avoid delays in the start of the study. If this is multiplied for each country, we can get a good idea of the complexity of the process.

The EC can terminate a clinical trial at any time if unanticipated problems come to light: if there is noncompliance with health authority regulations, especially those that jeopardize the safety of research subjects; for failure of the PI to report serious adverse events in a timely manner to the EC; and for an unacceptable standard of monitoring research subjects during the clinical trial by the PI.

Different countries have different rules regarding protecting the privacy of research subjects. The privacy rules are designed to safeguard the privacy of the research subject while ensuring medical information can be shared with medical professionals that are responsible for overseeing the medical care of the research subject. In the United

States the privacy rule is called the Health Insurance Portability and Accountability Act (HIPAA).

Institutional Biosafety Committees

Another type of committee may oversee biosafety at investigative sites for certain types of drugs that are experimental or biological in nature. In the United States, these committees are known as institutional biosafety committees. These committees review documentation provided by the sponsor that details the handling of any biological material that is used to make the drug. They may advise the pharmacy staff as well as the nursing and medical staff about how the material should be handled and if any precautions should be taken when handling or administering it.

Specialized Committees for Other Types of Drugs

Other specialized committees and advisory committees may be set up at institutions or at the national level in countries to advise regulatory authorities and the public about experimental drugs. These specialized committees and advisory committees will vary in name, but their goal will usually be to ensure that the safety of the research subject is protected, and that the field of research is advanced within appropriate ethical boundaries. An example of such a committee is the Recombinant DNA Advisory Committee (RAC), which oversees gene therapy research in the United States (see Chapter 9).

Ethical Conduct of Clinical Trials

4

I remember watching a film several years ago about a clinical trial that was carried out in the United States[1]. In the infamous Tuskegee experiments in the United States, a study was carried out without the knowledge of the subjects. Suffering from syphilis, the subjects were led to believe that they were under a course of treatment (Tuskegee Syphilis Study Legacy Committee, 1996). These people were denied treatment, even after effective treatment became available, as part of the experiment. During World War II, the Nazis also carried out abhorrent experiments on human beings (Spitz, 2005). Unfortunately, there are many examples since these events of man's inhumanity to man. As a result of decades of exposing people to unethical and unsafe research practices, regulations were written to protect the rights and welfare of human subjects (Chapter 3). They help to ensure that clinical trials are conducted to ethical standards. When they can, research subjects should educate themselves so that they can hold institutions conducting clinical trials to account and to ensure that their own rights, the rights of those that they care about, and the rights of human beings in general are protected during clinical research.

The Declaration of Helsinki and Ethical Conduct of Clinical Trials

The Declaration of Helsinki (World Medical Association, 1964) is an important document that outlines the principles of ethical conduct during clinical trials. It was passed by the World Medical Association in 1964, but it is accepted throughout the world as an international standard of ethical practice for research involving human subjects.[1] These standards involve the need to obtain a research subject's informed consent before the subject can be entered into a clinical trial. It also requires that all clinical research is reviewed and overseen by an independent team of ethical and scientific experts (i.e., the ethics committee). Ethical standards must be accompanied by rigorous scientific practices, and these standards must be implemented using good clinical practice (GCP), which we consider next.

Good Clinical Practice

Clinical investigators worldwide are expected to follow GCP, which is a standard for the design, conduct, performance, monitoring, auditing, recording, analysis, and reporting of clinical trials. Good clinical practice helps to safeguard research subjects and to ensure that the study is conducted ethically. Professionals involved in clinical trials should receive ongoing training in GCP. Clinical investigators write down or document how the clinical trial is carried out. They also write down or document all the results obtained during the clinical trial. The sponsor should monitor how the study is being conducted to ensure that GCP standards are being adhered to. After an application is submitted for approval, the regulatory authorities will inspect aspects of the work done to determine the extent to which it was carried out according to GCP standards and in accordance with the clinical protocols submitted in the application. The informed consent process is a crucial aspect of GCP and the Declaration of Helsinki.

Informed Consent Process

Before enrolling in a clinical trial or study, all participants must sign an informed consent form. Obtaining informed consent from a research subject is a process, not a one-time occurrence. You should not be rushed through this process or made to feel that you are wasting someone's time by asking questions. You should make your best effort to understand the risks and potential benefits before signing the informed consent form. To illustrate this point, we will consider William's story.

William's Story

William is 65 years old. He was diagnosed with prostate cancer about 3 weeks ago. He has just returned from a visit to the investigative site for a clinical trial involving a new drug for prostrate cancer. Naturally, he has been feeling very anxious about his health. He has had a good meeting with the principal investigator, whom he liked very much. The principal investigator explained the different aspects of the clinical trial to him and asked him to think about enrolling. William found it very difficult to listen to the investigator as he explained the details about the clinical trial; in fact, he did not ask any questions. He was given the informed consent form to review at home and was scheduled to return tomorrow for an assessment to determine if he should be enrolled in the clinical trial or be given alternative treatment. His wife was anxiously waiting when he returned home. After he had given her an update on the visit with the principal investigator, William sat down with the informed consent form and began to read it. He realized that he had not heard anything that the principal investigator had explained to him, and the information presented in the informed consent form was difficult to understand due to some of the terminology used. He put the informed consent form away to take with him to the meeting with the principal investigator on the following day.

Points to Consider

1. William is going through a very difficult time in his life. A cancer diagnosis is a crisis situation.

2. William is finding it difficult to understand unfamiliar scientific terminology.

3. Deciding to review the informed consent at home was a good decision. He may need to participate in several meetings with the principal investigator and to review the informed consent form several times before making a final decision on whether or not to take part in the clinical trial.

4. William went to the investigative site alone. It would be a good idea for him to bring his wife for company next time. She may be able to repeat the information that is presented to him when they are at home and to take notes as the principal investigator is talking to her husband.

5. It would be wise for William to ask for a patient advocate (see Chapter 6). He needs assistance sifting through the scientific information, and he is also under a lot of anxiety because of his cancer diagnosis. The advocate will help to ensure that he is making the best decision regarding participation in the clinical trial.

6. The patient advocate can assist William by creating a list of questions that he can ask the principal investigator.

7. The patient advocate can help William evaluate if the principal investigator is qualified to conduct the clinical research.

8. William will need to meet with the patient advocate throughout the clinical trial to assess any updates in the informed consent form that are provided to him for

signature. These updates will be provided to him as the safety profile of the drug under study is updated.

9. William should ensure that the principal investigator has no financial conflicts of interest before enrolling in the clinical trial.

Ideally, the informed consent process should allow for a full disclosure of what is known about the drug so that participants can make an informed decision about whether or not to participate in the clinical trial. The informed consent form cannot possibly contain all the information that is known about the drug because of the vastness of the volume of data that is available. Consequently, principal investigators (PIs), researchers, and sponsors make judgments about what to include in the informed consent form.

Although participants will sign the informed consent form, it is not a binding contract. Participants can decide to withdraw their participation at any time. After entering the clinical trial, it is appropriate to ask periodically for updates on the safety results for other participants in the clinical trial.

All research subjects must be provided with the following information during the informed consent process (International Conference on Harmonization Tripartite Guideline, 1996):

• That the clinical trial involves research. In other words, that they are considering entering a clinical trial
• The purpose of the clinical trial
• The trial treatment(s) and the probability for assignment to each treatment
• The trial procedures to be followed, including all invasive procedures
• The subject's responsibilities
• Those aspects of the trial that are experimental
• The reasonably foreseeable risks or inconveniences to the subject and, when applicable, to an embryo, fetus, or nursing infant

- The reasonably expected benefits. When there is no intended clinical benefit to the subject, the subject should be made aware of this.
- The alternative procedure(s) or course(s) of treatment that may be available to the research subject, as well as their important potential benefits and risks
- How a subject will be treated if he or she becomes injured or ill from the clinical trial, and who will pay for this treatment
- The anticipated prorated payment, if any, to the subject for participating in the trial
- The anticipated expenses, if any, to the subject for participating in the trial
- That the subject's participation in the trial is voluntary and that the subject may refuse to participate or withdraw from the trial, at any time, without penalty or loss of benefits to which the subject is otherwise entitled
- That the monitor(s), the auditor(s), the ethics committee, and the regulatory authority(ies) will be granted direct access to the subject's original medical records for verification of clinical trial procedures and data, without violating the confidentiality of the subject, and that signing the informed consent form authorizes this access
- That records identifying the subject will be kept confidential and, to the extent permitted by the applicable laws or regulations, will not be made publicly available. If the results of the trial are published, the subject's identity will remain confidential.
- That the subject or the research subject's legally acceptable representative will be informed in a timely manner if information becomes available that may be relevant to the subject's willingness to continue participation in the trial
- The person(s) to contact for further information regarding the trial and the rights of trial subjects, and whom to contact in the event of trial-related injury

- The foreseeable circumstances or reasons under which the subject's participation in the trial may be terminated
- The expected duration of the subject's participation in the trial
- The approximate number of subjects involved in the trial
- If the study involves an experimental drug
- A clear definition of which parts of the study are experimental
- Any possible side effects, adverse events, risks, or discomfort that a subject might experience
- The results of toxicological studies carried out in animals

Because the informed consent form is supposed to be written in language that a lay person can understand, you should ask for clarification of any scientific terms that you do not understand when you meet with the PI or sub-investigator. You should tell the PI if you have concerns about the way the form is written or have difficulty understanding it from a lay person's point of view. The form should be written in a type font that is easy to read.

For Phase I clinical trials, the informed consent form should contain a description of any pertinent animal studies that have been carried out with the drug, including any toxicology studies. These studies involve the administration of the drug to animals at much higher doses than will be given to humans in order to determine the likely adverse effects of the drug. The informed consent form should identify if the animals were harmed at these doses or if any animals died. If data from the animal studies are not included in the informed consent form, it would be appropriate to request a summary of this information.

In later phases, the informed consent form should at least briefly contain a description of any previous clinical trials that were conducted with the drug. It should describe the benefits observed, the side effects, and adverse events. While reading these descriptions in the informed consent document, you should make notes of any aspects about which you would like to receive more information. Sometimes the work that has been carried out is available in the published literature. The research staff can indicate where to locate these published reports, or they can provide copies to you.

A research subject should expect to have a main point of contact at the investigative site. This person should be available when you have questions and is usually listed within the informed consent form. It will normally be the PI, or the person who is responsible for the conduct of the study at the institution concerned. Additionally, the informed consent form will name a person to contact concerning your rights as a research subject and who to contact in the event of a research-related injury. However, there are certain types of information that researchers will not be able to disclose to you because this would invalidate the ongoing research. For instance, they must not reveal if you are receiving placebo, the standard treatment that is already on the market, or the drug that is being studied. Often the investigator will not know which research subjects are receiving placebo and which are receiving the drug. These studies are known as double-blind studies, since neither the subjects nor the researchers know who is receiving the drug under study. Keeping this information secret ensures that the study is carried out to high scientific standards. If the investigator suspects that the drug may be making you ill, the investigator will be able to find out if you are receiving the placebo or the drug, and then decide if it would be best to remove you from the study for safety reasons.

Those who run clinical trials are also required to share the medical records of the person taking part in the clinical trial with the company that is sponsoring the clinical trial and with regulatory authorities. When you sign the informed consent form you are effectively providing permission for your records to be reviewed in this way. During the clinical trial, your name and identifying information such as address will be replaced with a unique code. If a safety report must be prepared and submitted to the sponsor and health authorities, you will be known only by the code assigned and not by your name. If you are uncomfortable with other people seeing your medical records, you should not sign the informed consent form.

Some Considerations before Signing the Informed Consent Form

If you are undertaking a clinical trial that will offer treatment for your condition or disease, be sure to evaluate other treatment options outside the study as well. It is possible that an alternative medicine that is already on the market may be more appropriate for you than the drug being tested in the clinical trial.

You should also find out how any side effects will be treated. Determine who will pay for your treatment if you are injured during the course of the experimental clinical research. Will you be able to receive additional treatment to help you recover if you become ill during the clinical trial? Will you be expected to have adequate medical insurance to cover you for the treatment of any adverse events experienced during the clinical trial? Have other patients already enrolled in the clinical trial experienced side effects or adverse events? If so, how bad were they?

You should ask the investigator if your participation will prevent you from receiving available treatments in the future. Given the time required for study participation, the state of your health, or the stage of your disease, you should carefully weigh the benefits of joining a particular study. The riskier or more experimental the study, the more carefully you should consider your participation.

Participation in a clinical trial will require that you remain committed to participating in the clinical trial for the duration of the clinical trial. You should ensure that you will be able to attend follow-up meetings at the investigative site. The PI will monitor the effect of the drug on your body, so it is important to attend these meetings. Clinical trials have different durations depending on the study design and the disease for which the drug is being developed. For instance, because antibiotics are given for short periods of time, a study involving a new antibiotic may last only 10 to 14 days or even less. On the other hand, a study involving a treatment for a chronic illness like rheumatoid arthritis may last for 6 months, or longer.

Questions to Ask Yourself before Enrolling in a Clinical Trial

1. Do I know enough about this clinical trial to give informed consent?
2. What is expected of me?
3. Do I understand all the language used in the informed consent form?
4. Who is my main contact if I have questions or I am experiencing side effects (phone number, 24 hours contact number, etc.)?
5. How often will I need to attend appointments and see the investigator, and how will this affect my routine?
6. Am I clear on how often and how (before, with, or after food, etc.) to take the drug?
7. Will I be able to receive additional treatment to help me recover after an adverse event that may have been caused by the drug under study, at no cost to me?
8. Will I be expected to have adequate medical insurance to cover me for some aspects of the clinical trial?
9. Have other patients already enrolled in the clinical trial experienced side effects or adverse events? If so, how bad were they?

Questions to Ask Yourself after Enrolling in a Clinical Trial

1. Do I still know enough about the clinical trial to continue to give informed consent?
2. Is the mechanism for providing me with information about the safety profile from other research subjects in the study adequate?
3. Am I being kept adequately informed about the safety profile of the drug?
4. Have I been conscientious about reporting any adverse events and serious adverse events that I have experienced during this clinical trial?
5. Is this clinical trial still right for me?
6. Is the level of risk from this clinical trial still acceptable for my health?
7. Do I have enough understanding about new risks that have come to light since I enrolled in this clinical trial to make a decision on whether to continue in this clinical trial?
8. Am I comfortable with the level of oversight that is being given by the PI and other investigators to my care during this clinical trial?

Question to Ask the Principal Investigator after Enrolling in the Clinical Trial (See Other Questions in Chapter 7)

Have I signed the most up-to-date version of the informed consent document available?

Note

1. In the United States, the Belmont Report is an important document that identifies three fundamental ethical principles for all human subject research: respect

for persons, beneficence, and justice. Similar documents and reports may be available in other countries.

References

International Conference on Harmonization Tripartite Guideline. (1996). *Guideline for Good Clinical Practice E6(R1), Step 4 version*. http://www.ich.org/LOB/media/MEDIA482.pdf

Spitz, V. (2005). *Doctors from hell: The horrific account of Nazi experiments on humans*. Boulder, CO: Sentient.

Tuskegee Syphilis Study Legacy Committee. (1996). *Final Report of the Tuskegee Syphilis Study Legacy Committee. 1996-05-20*. Retrieved December 30, 2009, from http://www.hsl.virginia.edu/historical/medical_history/bad_blood/report.cfm

World Medical Association (WMA). (1964, June). *Declaration of Helsinki Ethical Principles for Medical Research Involving Human Subjects*. Adopted by the 18th WMA General Assembly, Helsinki, Finland, June.

————, and amended by the:

29th WMA General Assembly, Tokyo, Japan, October 1975

35th WMA General Assembly, Venice, Italy, October 1983

41st WMA General Assembly, Hong Kong, September 1989

48th WMA General Assembly, Somerset West, Republic of South Africa, October 1996 and the 52nd WMA General Assembly, Edinburgh, Scotland, October 2000

Note of Clarification on Paragraph 29 added by the WMA General Assembly, Washington 2002

Note of Clarification on Paragraph 30 added by the WMA General Assembly, Tokyo 2004.

55th WMA General Assembly, Seoul, 2008.

Assessing Risks versus Benefits

5

Two important documents help reduce risk and provide guidance in a clinical trial: the clinical protocol and the investigator's brochure. The clinical protocol is like a road map which describes how the clinical trial should be conducted. It states clearly who can be included in the clinical trial (inclusion criteria), who cannot be included (exclusion criteria), the side effects that must be watched for, the dosage of the drug, and the tests that will be carried out during the clinical trial. The investigator's brochure is another important document that is submitted to the ethics committee (EC) with the clinical protocol. The investigator's brochure describes the different aspects of the drug to be studied as well as the study procedures. It is written by the sponsor for the study staff. It describes how the animal experiments were carried out and how the results were obtained, as well as how the drug should be administered to the research subjects. It describes side effects and adverse events that may occur and how they can be recognized. It will also be submitted to the regulatory authority and

EC for review as part of the investigational new drug (IND) and clinical trial application processes.

What Are "Inclusion Criteria"?

The Glossary provides the meaning of jargon and terms that clinical trial staff use. Two terms that are often used are "inclusion criteria" and "exclusion criteria." These are criteria defined by the sponsor, agreed to by the principal investigator (PI) and sub-investigators, and written into the clinical protocol. To be accepted into a clinical trial, a subject must fit within certain criteria for that particular study. These are called inclusion criteria. Inclusion criteria serve as a checklist for those who decide if a patient should be accepted into a clinical trial. The checklist helps the medical professionals who are running the study to determine if a subject is a suitable candidate for the trial. Why is this necessary? The study's purpose is to learn how to treat a disease or condition. If a subject does not have the disease under study, he or she will not fit the inclusion criteria.

You must strive to be as truthful and forthcoming as you can about your own health. Those running the study will want to know what other treatments you are receiving or have received in the past, as well as details of your medical history, to ensure that the procedures and drugs that will be administered to you during the clinical trial will not harm you or cause dangerous drug–drug interactions.

What Are "Exclusion Criteria"?

Exclusion criteria are a checklist of requirements that automatically require that the PI exclude the research subject from participating in the clinical trial. Again, you must be truthful about your health, medical history, and any medicines that you are taking, so that it can be determined if you fit the exclusion criteria. If you have other accompanying diseases that may complicate the study, you may meet the criteria for exclusion. If you are not as healthy as you need to be to take part in the study, you may be excluded from taking part in the study.

You may be harmed if you are included in a clinical trial from which you should be excluded. There may be other clinical trials or treatments that are more appropriate for you or your condition. To illustrate the importance of revealing your complete medical history in your discussions with the PI and staff to determine if you are eligible for enrollment in a clinical trial, let's consider Martina's case.

Martina's Story

Martina is being treated for moderate depression, but she still experiences depressive episodes. She decided to take part in a clinical trial designed to test a new drug intended for moderate depression, but she chose not to mention that she was already taking an antidepressant in the monoamine oxidase inhibitor (MAOI) family of medicines; she had read in the informed consent document that this would exclude her from taking part in the clinical trial. Martina was accepted into the clinical trial. During her participation in the clinical trial, the drug being tested interacted with the MAOI and Martina had a very bad reaction. She was hospitalized and placed in the Intensive Care Unit. In going through Martina's medical history with her again, she divulged to the PI that she was taking a MAOI. The serious adverse event caused by the interaction was reported to the sponsor by the PI. The sponsor filed a safety report with the regulatory authority.

Points to Consider

1. Drug–drug interactions can be life threatening.
2. Martina risked her life by not disclosing that she was taking a MAOI.

3. Had Martina disclosed that she was taking this medicine, she would not have met the inclusion criteria for the study. She would have met the exclusion criteria and would not have been enrolled into the study. Her health would not have been compromised.

4. It is very important that research subjects inform the PI about all the medications they are taking, even over-the-counter medications.

5. It is not possible to know all the drug–drug interactions that might occur when a research subject takes a drug that is under study. The PI will note any drug–drug interactions so they can be documented quickly and conveyed to other investigators and subjects participating in the trial.

6. The sponsor and investigator will ensure that the information on drug–drug interactions is submitted to the regulatory authority.

The Phases of Clinical Development

The clinical trial process is divided into phases: Phase 1, Phase 2, Phase 3, and Phase 4. It is crucial that a seriously ill patient understands the difference between an experimental drug that is being studied in a Phase 1 clinical trial and an already registered medicine being studied during a Phase 4 clinical trial. We will therefore take some time to explain the differences between the phases and illustrate the differences with some fictional stories.

Each medicine that is approved by regulatory authorities has usually gone through three main phases of drug development: Phase 1, Phase 2, and Phase 3. Studies carried out after the medicine is on the market are usually termed "Phase 4 studies" if they are carried out according to the approved product label and "Phase 3 studies" if they are not carried out strictly in accordance with the approved product information. Phase 4 studies are carried out on a marketed medicine to find out more about the medicine in the real-life situation than could be learned during the clinical trials.

Several clinical trials will usually be carried out during each phase of drug development. Sometimes more than one phase may be ongoing at the same time. In Phase 1, researchers study a small number of healthy volunteers (approximately 100 to 200 subjects). These are people who do not usually have the disease that the medicine is eventually expected to treat. Researchers try to determine the appropriate dosage of a drug, or the frequency of administration that should be followed. Although Phase 1 studies are often carried out in healthy volunteers, if the drug is intended to treat a serious illness such as cancer, they will usually only be carried out in patients with the disease. A Phase 1 study that is carried out in patients should be regarded as experimental, meaning that there is usually no proof at this stage that the drug works. Patients should not enter such a clinical trial with the expectation that their disease will be cured or even treated. The chances of this happening in Phase 1 are lower than during a late-stage Phase 3 study after efficacy has been demonstrated during earlier phases, or a Phase 4 study.

Phase 1 clinical trials involve researching how the drug is metabolized (broken down by the body). The design of the Phase 1 study may include a control group of healthy volunteers that takes either a placebo (no actual drug is present) or a medicine that is already available on the market. To illustrate some of the principles of Phase 1 studies, we would like to introduce you to Dominic, who is a postgraduate student at a university.

Dominic's Story

Dominic is a postgraduate student at a local university. One day he was having lunch with Tom, a friend, who is a physician who treats patients with asthma. Tom was running a Phase 1 clinical trial to test the use of inhalers filled with an inert placebo powder. The purpose of this clinical trial is to determine if the inhaler device delivers sufficient placebo powder into the lungs and could be used to deliver respiratory medicines. Tom described the requirements for participation in the study over lunch and asked Dominic if he would like to participate. The study would require that Dominic test the mechanics of the inhaler and write down his findings. He would also note any side effects he experienced. A small amount of money would be paid for his participation. Dominic believed that it would be a good use of his time to participate and so he agreed to meet with Tom in his office later that afternoon to enroll into the clinical trial.

Points to Consider

1. This is a healthy volunteer study, otherwise known as a Phase 1 clinical trial.
2. The risks of the clinical research in this specific situation are relatively low, but not nonexistent; the clinical trial involves the inhalation of a placebo powder. Dominic might experience an allergic reaction or problems with breathing while testing the inhaler. This risk must be considered before signing the informed consent form.
3. Dominic may have been motivated to participate in the clinical trial by the money he would be paid for his participation. The amount to be paid for his participation is not supposed to be sufficient to induce him to take part in the clinical trial.
4. In approaching a friend to take part in this clinical trial, Tom must avoid placing him under an obligation to take part. Likewise, Dominic should not feel pressured to agree to enroll in the clinical trial because he was asked to participate by someone that he knows well.

In Phase 2, investigators may run clinical trials, in several hundred research subjects with the disease that the drug is eventually intended to treat. The main goal of Phase 2 studies is to find an appropriate dose that may lead to efficacy and to determine the best patient group in which to study the drug. The efficacy of the drug is examined during Phase 2 clinical trials. These studies are often randomized. Randomization means that patients are assigned to a group by chance—this is like tossing a coin and deciding into which group a patient should be placed. Some patients may receive the drug, while others may receive a placebo which contains no drug, or a comparator drug that is already approved and marketed. The goal of randomized placebo-controlled studies is to ensure that any efficacy observed during a clinical trial is a real effect and did not occur by chance. Extensive information on safety and efficacy are collected on patients who receive the placebo as well as those who receive the drug under study. This enables researchers to see if the drug is causing adverse events and serious adverse events. Open label studies are those that are not conducted with a control group. They are also not randomized. Researchers and research subjects will usually know which treatments are being administered. To illustrate some of the principles of Phase 2 studies, we will review Bridget's experience.

Bridget's Story

Bridget suffers from severe systemic lupus erythematosus (lupus), which is not adequately controlled on medications that are available. The hospital specialist that is treating her suggested that she enter a Phase 2 study ongoing at the hospital to find a suitable dose for a possible new treatment for lupus. She agreed to join the study because although she would be able to continue on her current treatments, there would be a possibility to experience efficacy. Bridget is not sure which dose she will receive after joining the study. She is currently reviewing the informed consent form and making a list of questions to ask the PI when she meets with her later that afternoon.

Points to Consider

Some questions that Bridget may want to ask the PI are as follows:

1. How many other dose groups have been studied so far?
2. How many patients are entered into each group?
3. Have any serious adverse events been observed so far?
4. What were the target organs in the animal studies?
5. Have the same organs been impacted in humans as in the animal toxicology studies?
6. Have any research subjects been removed from the study due to safety concerns? If yes, did the safety issues resolve with time after the research subjects were removed from the study?
7. If I am injured in this clinical trial, how will any treatment that I need be paid for?
8. Can you think of other questions that Bridget should consider asking?

In the United States, a special one-off meeting is held with the Food and Drug Administration (FDA) called an End of Phase 2 Meeting, at which the FDA will review the results from previous phases and, if appropriate, give approval for Phase 3 to commence. If not appropriate at that point, the FDA could ask the company to conduct additional Phase 2 or even Phase 1 studies. In other countries, meetings can be held with health authorities at any time and may have less proscribed timetables.

In Phase 3, several thousand people may participate in clinical trials and receive the drug already studied in the previous two phases. The size of Phase 3 studies is dependent on the disease and the patient group in which it occurs. For instance, a Phase 3 program for a very rare disease may consist of only 20 research subjects, while a Phase 3 program for an antidepressant may consist of several thousand research subjects. Depending on the duration of the treatment and follow-up stages of the Phase 3 studies, Phase 3 may stretch over several years to determine any long-term effects of the drug, or last only 3 to 6 months. Duration is an important factor in disease, and these requirements are set by regulatory authorities on the basis of scientific understanding of the disease and the ability of the clinical research process to predict for the real-life situation. To gain an understanding of the concepts involved with Phase 3 studies, we will consider Maria's story.

Maria's Story

Maria is a 40-year-old science teacher with severe rheumatoid arthritis. Her disease is very debilitating and is not controlled on current treatments. Her general practitioner has advised her of a Phase 3 clinical trial of a drug that showed good results during Phase 2 clinical trials. If the two ongoing Phase 3 studies show good results, the sponsor will most likely be able to secure a regulatory approval to market the drug. Maria's general practitioner suggested that she meet with the PI to discuss taking part in the clinical trial. He is particularly eager for her to enroll in the clinical trial because the drug has shown good results in patients who are not well controlled on currently available medicines.

Points to Consider

1. This is a Phase 3 study for a drug that has already shown good results in earlier studies.
2. Maria's rheumatoid arthritis is not currently controlled with her medication. Presuming she meets the inclusion/exclusion criteria, this clinical trial might be able to provide benefit to Maria.

After a medicine is approved by health authorities such as the FDA, and the medicine is on the market, it may be studied further in Phase 4. These studies have the goal of finding the best use for the medicine in much larger patient populations than was possible in the clinical trials that were conducted before marketing.

Table 5.1 Comparison of Phase 1, 2, 3 and 4 Studies

	Description	No. of Research Subjects
Phase 1	Early studies to determine the effect of the therapeutic on the body	20 to 80 subjects per clinical trial
	Low dose levels are studied, usually in healthy volunteers.	Each Phase 1 clinical trial can last from several days to several weeks.
	Different dose schedules can be studied during Phase 1	
	Several clinical trials will be carried out in Phase 1.	
	The therapeutic may be administered to humans for the first time.	
	Patients are enrolled in Phase 1 studies if they have a serious disease and the risk–benefit profile cannot justify administering the therapeutic to a healthy research subject.	
Phase 2	Phase 2 studies are carried out in patients.	100 to 250 patients may be included in a typical Phase 2 study.
	Phase 2 studies are divided into Phase 2A or early studies and Phase 2B studies	
	Phase 2A studies are used to determine the appropriate dose to be given to patients. The starting doses may have been studied during Phase 1 clinical trials.	
	The Phase 2 studies will often involve the administration of placebo and therapeutic agents to different groups of patients.	
Phase 3	These are longer and larger studies that seek to reproduce the situation that the therapeutic is being developed to treat.	300 to 3000 patients may be included in a typical Phase 3 study.
	These studies are designed to determine whether the therapeutic is effective, and if it is safe.	
	Side effects that occur after administration.	
Phase 4	The objective of these studies is to learn more about the therapeutic in the real-life situation.	These studies can include hundreds of patients or many thousands.
	These studies can also include trials of different doses or schedules of administration, other stages of disease or other disease and age groups, cost studies, quality-of-life studies, or use of the drug over a longer period of time than was studied during the clinical trials before the drug was registered.	

The approved medicine may also be studied in different diseases from those for which it was registered. As mentioned previously, these studies may be considered Phase 3 studies if they are outside of the registered product label.

The different phases of clinical trial study are shown in Table 5.1.

The Risk–Benefit Ratio

The balance of risk and benefit is a very important concept for those taking part in clinical trials and for those overseeing them. The potential for benefit increases as the program moves from Phase 1 to Phase 3. A risk–benefit ratio is like a scale (Fig. 5.1). As you can see from Figure 5.1, on one side of the scale is risk, and on the other side of the scale is benefit. The challenge is to ensure that there is sufficient balance between risk and benefit and that the scales are tipped further onto the side of benefit than onto the side of risk. When the risk outweighs the benefit, this is not considered to be good for those who are taking part in the clinical trial.

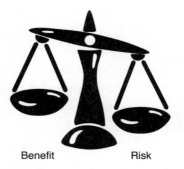

Benefit   Risk

Figure 5.1 Risk-benefit analysis is similar to a set of scales.

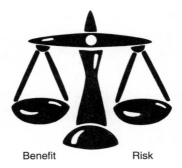

Benefit   Risk

Figure 5.2 A balance of risks and benefits is the ideal situation.

The goal is to have a balance between risk and benefit (Fig. 5.2). In Figure 5.2, risk and benefit are equal. In some situations, risks may be acceptable even if they outweigh the benefits because a patient may be suffering from a life-threatening illness, and this trial may have the potential to help the patient. When a drug is likely to, or known to have too many risks, for instance, if it is intended to be studied for the treatment of cancer, the Phase 1 studies must be carried out in patients rather than healthy volunteers. In this situation the drug has too much risk to be administered to healthy volunteers. In these situations, by giving the drug to patients, the risks are better balanced out with an eventual potential benefit. Research subjects should ask questions that enable them to establish the risk–benefit ratio for their particular situation, and to assess whether the balance is acceptable to them or not, before participating in a clinical trial.

During Phase 2, researchers continue to modify and refine the research methods to reflect the new information gained from ongoing clinical research. If the drug proves beneficial at this stage and outweighs the risks or side effects, then the development moves to Phase 3.

Adverse Events and Serious Adverse Events

Ensuring the safety of research subjects during a clinical trial is crucial. No drug is completely safe. The level of safety will depend on the dose that is given to the patient and the reaction that the patient's body has to it. Therefore, it is very important that the research subject is observed closely after the drug is administered during a clinical trial. Side effects and adverse events may occur after a drug is administered. A side effect is a by-product or result of the drug's pharmacological activity in the body. For instance an antihypertensive drug may have the potential for development of hypotension as a side effect. An adverse event is any adverse outcome that occurs within a reasonable timeframe of giving the drug, even if it is not caused by the drug under study. By analyzing the adverse events that occur after a drug is administered, it may be possible to work out which adverse events may be caused by the drug, which may be caused by the disease, and which may have occurred by coincidence.

Pharmaceutical companies and investigators must report adverse events to regulatory authorities within strict deadlines. Adverse events that occur during a clinical trial are reported to the sponsor, the health authorities, and to the EC. If the adverse event is not serious, it can be reported less quickly. Rapid reporting gives the regulatory authority time to respond and to intervene in the clinical trial if necessary. This intervention may involve the termination of the study so that additional research subjects cannot enter the clinical trial. The intervention may also involve changing the clinical protocol to make the clinical trial safer.

Principal investigators are required to report adverse events that are serious, unexpected, and associated with the drug being studied. When a serious adverse event occurs that is unexpected and associated with the drug under study, this adverse event must be reported to the regulatory authority within 15 days. It must be reported to the regulatory authority within 7 days if it is life threatening. For studies that are ongoing abroad, unexpected serious adverse or life-threatening adverse events must be reported to all other countries conducting studies with the drug within 15 days of the sponsor receiving notice that the related serious adverse event has occurred. In order for these reporting requirements to be met, sponsors will usually define which adverse events and serious events should be reported to them in an expedited manner by the investigator to give them time to file the report to the regulatory authorities.

Investigators often use terms such as *not related, possibly related, probably related,* or *definitely related* when speaking about adverse events. These terms relate to the level of certainty that can be assigned that the adverse event or serious adverse event was caused by the drug. The assignment of the degree of certainty is also known as a *causality assignment.* Figure 5.3 shows the level of certainty attached to the terms *not related, possibly related, probably related,* and *definitely related.* There is a greater amount of certainty for a "definite" causality assignment than for a "possible" causality assignment. There is also a good amount of certainty for a "not related" causality assignment.

Definitely Related	↑	Highest level of certainty
Probably Related		
Possibly Related		Low level of certainty
Not Related/Unrelated		High level of certainty

Figure 5.3 Schematic showing the level of certainty assigned that an adverse event or serious adverse event is related to the investigational agent.

We close this chapter with some questions about risks and benefits that you may wish to ask yourself, the pharmacist and the PI before you enroll in a clinical trial, as well as questions to ask the PI after you have enrolled in the clinical trial. Some questions to ask your medical insurance provider are also included.

Questions to Ask Yourself before Enrolling in a Clinical Trial

1. Do I understand the potential adverse events and side effects that I might experience during this clinical trial?
2. Is this the best clinical trial for me to take part in?
3. Given what I know about this clinical trial, is there an acceptable risk to my health?
4. Do I understand enough about the potential risks to make a decision on whether or not to take part in this clinical trial?
5. Does the clinical trial involve research of an unproven or experimental drug?
6. What is the purpose of the clinical research?
7. How long is the clinical trial expected to last?
8. Are there any procedures that will cause discomfort or put my health at risk?
9. What are the possible benefits to me of my participation in this clinical trial?
10. Are there any procedures or treatments that would be more appropriate for me to consider than this clinical trial?
11. Will I need to be admitted into the hospital during the clinical trial?
12. Who will provide my medical care after the clinical trial ends?
13. Who will provide my medical care if I am terminated from this clinical trial after enrolling?

14. Should I stop my current medication after starting the clinical trial?
15. Will my medical insurance company need to pay toward the costs of the clinical trial?

Questions to Ask a Pharmacist before Enrolling in a Clinical Trial

The following questions can be discussed with your pharmacist. Ensure that you provide the pharmacist with the informed consent form and any additional information on the clinical trial that you have received from the investigative site.

1. From a review of my medical history and the over-the-counter and prescribed medications I take, would I be at risk of drug–drug interactions by taking part in this clinical trial?
2. Is there any information concerning my current medications about which I should inform the principal investigator?
3. Can you provide me with a printout of my medication history to provide to the PI?

Questions to Ask the Principal Investigator before Enrolling in the Clinical Trial

1. What sorts of serious adverse events might I experience during my participation in the clinical trial?
2. What types of toxicities were experienced by the animals during the good laboratory practice toxicology studies?
   a. To what extent are these toxicities expected to occur in research subjects?
   b. To what extent are these toxicities not relevant at the doses that I will be administered during the clinical trial?

Questions to Ask the Principal Investigator after Enrolling in the Clinical Trial

1. Has any new safety or efficacy information come to light since I enrolled in the clinical trial that was not known when I signed the informed consent document?
2. Is this still the best study for me?
3. What phase of the clinical trial are we currently in? (Phase 1, 2, 3, or 4)
4. What phase of the clinical trial is the drug currently in? (Phase 1, 2, 3, or 4)
5. Have there been any deaths in the clinical trial after my participation? If yes, were any of these deaths considered related to the drug under study?
6. Have any animals died during additional toxicological studies since I joined the clinical trial? If yes, has the safety margin for the medicine been reduced? Has this information been added to a revised informed consent form? If yes, when will I be able to review the new informed consent form?

Questions to Ask the Principal Investigator after Completing Participation in a Clinical Trial

If you are experiencing adverse events that occurred after your participation in a clinical trial, it is appropriate to bring these to the attention of the PI. The PI can decide whether or not to report them to the sponsor.

1. Could this adverse event that I have been experiencing be related to the drug that was administered during the clinical trial?
2. Who will reimburse my medical expenses that have resulted from this adverse event?
3. What do you recommend I do now to preserve my health?

Questions to Ask the Medical Insurance Provider

1. If I am injured in this clinical trial, will my insurance cover my treatments?
2. Will the insurance coverage be provided until I am completely recovered? If not, to what extent will I be covered?

Other Issues to Consider as a Research Subject

6

About 2 years ago I attended a meeting with a client company. We were looking forward to hearing the presentation by a corporate physician who had been involved with the development of a life-saving drug for a difficult-to-treat cancer. The meeting was being held at a patient advocacy group facility. The speaker described some of the challenges that the company had faced in developing the drug and how they had been overcome; then he asked if there were any questions. Sitting next to me was a woman who told the speaker that her husband was being treated with a drug that was under study. As she began to talk about the clinical trial that her husband was enrolled in, my clients and I realized that this happened to be the drug that my client company was developing. I could sense her anxiety mixed with hope. It brought home to me just how much hope research subjects and their families place in clinical research.

What's in It for Me?

People enroll in clinical trials for many different reasons. Some of these reasons are as follows:

- A healthy student may volunteer to take part in a clinical trial because the research may help patients with the disease that will be studied.
- A patient with cancer may have been advised that there are no other treatment options, but that there are ongoing clinical trials that should be considered.
- A patient that is terminally ill may have heard that there have been some good responses in an ongoing clinical trial.
- A parent may decide that a clinical trial is an appropriate option for a young child because it might help researchers to find out more about how to treat the rare disease that the child is suffering from.
- A patient that is terminally ill may decide to take part in a clinical trial involving a new, but experimental approach with the hope that taking part in the clinical trial may help others with the disease.
- Regular and thorough checkups and free medication may be some of the benefits of participation in a clinical trial. Payments for participation in clinical trials are set to ensure that people are not induced into taking part in trials by receiving large payments. Nevertheless, some people may wrongly seek to enter clinical trials in order to receive payments for participation.

These are only some examples of the reasons why people decide to take part in clinical trials. Let's review Jack's reasons for wanting to take part in a clinical trial.

Jack's Story

Jack is a 19-year-old university student who is studying physiology. While on the bus to the university campus a few days ago, he

heard a radio announcement about an opportunity for healthy
volunteers to enroll in a clinical trial to test a novel treatment for
hypertension. Upon arriving at the campus he logged onto the
Internet and found the Web site for the clinical research organiza-
tion that was conducting the clinical study. He decided to give
them a call to find out more. He is in excellent health and believes
that he will almost certainly meet any criteria for inclusion.
He particularly wanted to find out how much money he would be
paid for taking part in the clinical trial. A while ago he had heard
some of his friends say that participation in clinical trials could pay
quite well. He is behind in paying for his university tuition and
this would be a way to catch up.

Points to Consider

1. Jack's motivation is purely financial for taking part in a
   clinical trial as a healthy volunteer. Clinical trial stipends
   must be set so as not to be an inducement to people
   like Jack who are in need of money for many different
   reasons.
2. Jack's financial situation is likely to influence his decision on whether to enroll in the clinical trial. His
   judgment about whether this is a good clinical trial for
   him is likely to be clouded by his financial concerns.
3. Jack is in good health, but he should review the information on the clinical trial carefully to ensure that participation in it will not put his excellent health at risk.

Should I Join a Clinical Trial?

When considering whether to join a clinical trial, you may find it
helpful to consider what *you* hope to achieve by taking part. Whatever
your reason for choosing to take part in a trial, you will want to weigh
the requirements as well as the amount of time and energy that it

will take for you to participate. Never feel pressured to take part in a clinical trial. Even if you are told that there are no other treatments available, take the time to evaluate the pros and cons of the clinical trial that is offered to you. If you decide not to participate in the clinical trial, your physician is required to offer you alternative forms of treatment for your illness or condition.

How Can I Find a Suitable Clinical Trial?

If you are interested in taking part in a clinical trial, there are a number of methods that you can use to find a suitable one:

- The Internet is a useful tool for finding clinical trials. If you are unfamiliar with how to use the Internet, a librarian at a public library will be able to offer you some assistance. Chapter 14 provides a useful list of Web sites that you can consult to locate possible clinical trials.
- Patient advocacy and support groups are a good source of information on ongoing clinical trials. Chapter 14 lists some of the patient advocacy groups that you may find helpful. The list provided is not exhaustive. Others can be found on the Internet or by visiting your local library.
- You can find clinical trials that are listed in your geographical area by doing an Internet search. Type in your town or state and "clinical trials," "medical testing," or "clinical trial participants needed," and the disease or illness that you are suffering from.
- Radio stations will sometimes advertise for healthy volunteers and patients for clinical trials.
- Pharmaceutical company Web sites will provide details about ongoing clinical trials.
- You can ask your doctor for clinical trial recommendations. Your doctor is likely to hear of ongoing clinical trials by reading medical

journals and from attendance at conferences and meetings, and he or she may be able to suggest clinical trials that are suitable for you. Your doctor may also be able to refer you to the physicians or a hospital where suitable clinical trials are being conducted.

- Call university hospitals in your area to learn if they are running any suitable clinical trials. You can also visit http://www.clinicaltrials.gov (for studies in the United States) and search by disease or condition, by funding organization, and by type of research subject sought. Before contacting the institution mentioned, discuss if the clinical trial is suitable for you with your general practitioner.

What Do I Need to Do to Participate in a Clinical Trial?

The PI or sub-investigator will take a detailed medical history from you. The study may require the healthy functioning of particular body organs (e.g., your kidneys or your liver). For most clinical trials, you will be given a full medical examination, including the taking of blood to determine if you qualify for participation in the clinical trial. These examinations will be carried out on all research subjects, healthy volunteers as well as patients. The purpose of the examination is to find out what your health was like before you entered the clinical trial. This makes it possible to determine what effect the drug may have on your body.

What Are My Obligations as a Research Subject?

Your job as a research subject is to follow the directions that are given to you by the PI. These directions will have been taken from the clinical protocol. For instance, it will be important for you to attend the visits to meet with the PI or sub-investigators at the appropriate times according to the clinical protocol so that the PI can see if the drug is causing unseen adverse events or is having a beneficial effect on your disease. Alternatively, if you are asked to write down your experience with the drug in a patient diary on a daily basis, or to take a certain number of tablets or capsules daily, it will be important to comply with these instructions. If you do not follow the PI's directions, you could put your health at risk or affect the overall results of the clinical trial. If you consistently fail to follow instruction, you may be terminated from further participation in the study.

What Is an Experimental Drug?

The term *experimental* implies that the drug or approach is cutting edge or novel and therefore unproven. You should carefully consider taking part in a clinical trial involving an experimental approach or drug if you are terminally ill or if you do not have many treatment options. The process of being informed about an experimental drug is more difficult because there may not be a lot known about its potential to cause benefit or to inflict harm.

What Should I Tell My Family and Close Friends?

When entering a clinical trial, it is appropriate to make your family and close friends aware of your participation. The hospital or institution that is running the clinical trial should ask you for contact details for someone who can be called in the event that you experience a medical emergency during the trial.

What Is a Patient Advocate?

Patient advocates work in many major hospitals, clinics, and hospices. It is possible that the number of such individuals may not meet the demand, especially in difficult economic times. Even if you are not allocated a patient advocate, you can ask someone close to you to play that role.

As the name indicates, patient advocates represent a patient and his or her best interests. An advocate is crucial for research subjects that do not have control over their faculties or whose memory, mental state, or physical state is severely impaired. They can also be very helpful if you feel overwhelmed by the amount or complexity of information that is being given to you. They can sift through the information with you and help you to determine what is best for your health and personal situation. They can even accompany you to your visits to see the investigator and assist you with asking questions. An advocate is someone who is confident about speaking to clinical trial professionals. Ask to be assigned a patient advocate if you feel you need one.

If you are seriously ill, it is normal for you to experience many different and often very disturbing emotions. People who are seriously ill will naturally worry about whether they will get better. They may be in a lot of pain or may be worried about the impact of their disease on family members. Under these circumstances, a sick person may find it difficult to focus on important information that is being shared by the investigator or study nurse. An advocate will listen to the information and ask the questions that need to be asked. The patient advocate will carefully take notes and then review everything with the patient that was explained by the investigator.

Although advocates are often associated with the investigative site, you are free to bring your own representative to act as your advocate. An advocate may be a lay person, a pastor or minister, a family member, a friend, or someone who is a physician or an attorney.

The Role of the Clinical Investigator

Because clinical trials involve the study of disease, physicians play an important role in them. The principal investigator (PI) is the person in charge of medical oversight of the clinical trial. The investigators that work under the supervision of the PI are called sub-investigators. The PI and sub-investigators are sometimes referred to generically as clinical investigators. Clinical investigators conduct clinical research within their hospitals, clinics, and offices. These locations are often referred to as investigative or investigational sites. Besides being medically qualified, clinical investigators must also have specialist expertise and knowledge about treating the disease that is being studied. This chapter will provide you with information about the clinical investigators, in order to prepare you for your meetings with them.

In the United States, physicians can apply to the Food and Drug Administration (FDA) to conduct their own clinical trials. These are known as physician-initiated investigational new drug applications (INDs).[1] These studies are regarded by some as less rigorously conducted than the industry-sponsored clinical trials. If you are a patient, you should try to find out if the research is conducted under a corporate-sponsored IND or a physician-sponsored IND. If the physician is conducting the clinical research under a physician-sponsored IND, it would be appropriate to determine the physician's purpose in conducting the research, the source of the drug that will be studied in the clinical trial, and what will be done with the results after they are collected.

The PI is the person you may see regularly when you make your visits to the investigative site during the clinical trial. You may also see one or more of the sub-investigators during study visits, as well as study nurses, study coordinators, pharmacists, laboratory staff, and others involved in the running of the study. Clinical investigators administer the drug under study and write down the results on special forms known as case report forms (CRFs).

Most importantly, the PI is responsible for ensuring the safety and welfare of research subjects during the clinical trial. The PI and sub-investigators must also document any efficacy or signs that the drug is curing the disease on the CRF. The PI should be available to meet with you and answer questions, with appropriate notice. During a clinical trial, there are many competing interests. The PI provides the check and balance. For instance, the PI may require that a participant's enrollment in a study be terminated if it is clear that it is no longer in the best interest of the research subject to continue in the clinical trial. The PI may also decide that a particular research subject would be best served by taking part in another clinical trial or by being removed from the clinical trial in order to receive treatment that is already approved.

There must be an appropriate separation of the responsibilities between the sponsor of the study and the PI/sub-investigators. Investigators that believe that the sponsor is interfering with their relationship with their patients can file a complaint with the ethics committee (EC) and the regulatory authority. The EC and the regulatory authority may decide to investigate the complaint and can sanction the sponsor and even prevent the individuals involved as well as the sponsor from conducting further clinical research. That said, it is important that the PI seeks permission from the sponsor before making changes to the clinical protocol. The only exception to this is if there is a safety reason to immediately make the change without seeking the sponsor's permission. The reason for this is that there are often many investigators at different investigative sites involved in each clinical trial. If all investigators made changes without seeking permission from the sponsor, the investigative sites would all be following different clinical protocols, and it would not be possible to gather meaningful results. Consequently, if a change is made at one investigative site, other investigators must also follow the changed protocol. Before the changed protocol can be implemented, it must be approved by the regulatory authority and the EC at each investigative site. Likewise, when the sponsor makes a change to the protocol, all investigators must follow the new protocol after it has been approved by the local EC and the regulatory authority.

Investigators that are involved in clinical trials will usually have other clinical duties within the institution. They may be seeing patients in clinics and on the wards for which they are responsible. Sometimes the PI will be a world-renowned physician. In this situation the sub-investigators often see the patients at the routine clinical trial visits. But PIs should still review the patient's information, even if they are unable to see the patient very often. You should raise questions if you have never been seen by a clinical investigator. The PI is responsible for making sure that the study is run according to local, national, and international regulations, with the best interests of the research subjects in mind. The PI also has the responsibility to ensure that the clinical research team follows the clinical protocol as it is written.

The sub-investigators report to the PI, who ensures that each participant is evaluated at each stage of the clinical trial to find out if participation continues to serve that subject's best interest. Sometimes a clinical trial participant may experience changes in health during the clinical trial. The PI may inform the research subject that he or she is being terminated from the study in these situations. If this happens to you, this does not mean that you have failed in your participation in the study. The PI will explain the other treatment options that are available to you or may suggest that you consider participation in an alternative clinical trial.

The PI or the sub-investigators will meet with the research subject at regular study visits to look for adverse events and serious adverse events. As explained in Chapter 5, the monitoring of the research subject for adverse events and serious adverse events is a critical aspect of ensuring research subjects' safety during clinical trials. When serious adverse events are observed to have occurred or to be in the process of occurring, the investigator must report them to the sponsor within appropriate timelines, and action must be taken with respect to the research subject to ensure that any harm is minimized.

Is My Principal Investigator Qualified to Conduct This Clinical Trial?

Many people are deferential and timid when it comes to dealing with physicians. However, you should not feel too intimidated to request information from the PI in charge of your clinical trial. You need to assure yourself that those conducting the clinical trial are qualified to do so. For example, a physician that is qualified and board certified to treat patients with respiratory diseases should not be acting as an investigator in a clinical trial for patients with cardiovascular disease.

Such a physician would not be qualified to provide the oversight for the research subjects in the study.

As a research subject or a potential research subject you are justified in asking to see credentials and specific information about the investigators in charge of and involved in the clinical trial in which you are considering participating. In particular, you should ask for any publications or papers that the investigators have written in the area of clinical research concerned. It is also appropriate for you to search the Internet for evidence that the PI is an expert in the area of study. If you do not have access to a computer, you can request help for this search from the librarian at your local library. You can check a Web site that contains research publications, known as PubMed (http://www.pubmed.com), a service of the National Library of Medicine, to see if the investigator has published any papers in the area of clinical research that you are considering. If you are unable to find any publications by the PI in the area of clinical research, ask the PI about his or her clinical research experience in this clinical area. Investigators involved with running clinical trials expect research subjects to ask questions. Just as you are interviewed to see if you are suitable for participation in a study, you should also treat your time with the investigators as an opportunity to interview *them*. Let's see how Solomon is considering handling this type of situation.

Solomon's Story

Solomon is a 65-year-old man who has been referred by his general practitioner to a dermatologist who is conducting a clinical trial on a new drug for the treatment of psoriasis, a disease of the skin. Solomon is currently being treated with immunosuppressants, but his disease has not been controlled adequately. He is someone who has been brought up to believe that physicians should be revered. He is preparing for his meeting at the investigative site and is making a list of questions to ask about the clinical trial.

Points to Consider

1. Solomon is concerned about appearing disrespectful if he raises questions during his visit with the investigator. The investigator should not view his questioning as disrespectful, but should welcome this as a sign that the research subject is interested in the study.
2. Solomon is making a list of questions in advance of his meeting with the investigator. This will enable Solomon to feel prepared for the meeting.
3. Since his general practitioner recommended the clinical trial to him, the general practitioner may also be able to help him to identify the important questions to ask the investigator.

Payment of Investigators

The investigative site is usually paid by the sponsor for its participation in clinical trials. The sponsor and the PI agree to a budget for the clinical trials. The sponsor usually pays the investigative site an amount on a per-research-subject basis. These monies are used to defray the costs of the study and will also contribute to the profit made by the institution at the end of the year. The payment arrangements are defined in a contract that may be reviewed as part of a clinical trial application by some regulatory authorities. The amounts paid per research subject will vary depending on the complexity of the clinical trial. For example, an outpatient study to evaluate a pain reliever may be less expensive to run on a per-research-subject basis than a study that involves in-hospital stays as well as many procedures and evaluations. The difference in the amounts to be paid will depend on the number of procedures to be carried out during the clinical trial and their complexity. A clinical trial in which research subjects must remain in the hospital for the clinical trial for any period of time will be more costly than a clinical trial in which the research subjects remain in their homes for the duration of the clinical trial.

What Does "Conflict of Interest" Mean?

Investigators that are involved in clinical trials should avoid financial conflicts of interest. A conflict of interest arises when the investigator has a financial interest in the outcome of the study. As examples of situations where this situation can occur, consider the following: the investigator owns a large equity stake in the company that is sponsoring the study; the investigator is the sponsor of the study, and will gain commercially if it is successful; or the investigator is the owner of the company that is sponsoring the study. Determining a conflict of interest is very important for several reasons. If someone with a financial conflict of interest personally conducts a clinical trial, there is a greater perceived temptation for that person to influence the outcome of the clinical trial to his or her financial advantage than if that person had no financial interest. Ideally, ECs should ensure that you are informed of any conflict of interests the PI may have so that you can make a truly informed decision about participating in a clinical trial. Because this may not always occur, depending on local rules and national regulations and guidelines, you should raise the question with the PI if this information is absent from the informed consent form. Consider asking the following questions:

- Who is funding this study?
- Do you have any ownership interest in the drug that is under study?
- Do you have a financial or ownership interest in the company that is sponsoring this study?

Investigators with a large equity interest in a sponsor company should be limited in their direct involvement in a clinical trial involving your treatment or granting of informed consent. However, the extent to which such an investigator may be permitted to treat you during the clinical trial may depend on national regulations and local investigative site guidelines. Appropriately, other investigators should take on the active day-to-day work of the clinical research in these situations.

In the United States,[2] the FDA has issued Part 54 under the Code of Federal Regulations (2008) to guide investigators, investigational sites, and sponsors to avoid financial conflicts of interest. Part 54 and the guideline (U.S. Department of Health and Human Services, 2001) requires that sponsors identify and notify the FDA in the final marketing application if any investigators that took part in the clinical studies had a proprietary interest in the product that was tested. This can include a patent, copyright, trademark, or a licensing agreement. The sponsor is also required to notify the FDA if any investigators had a significant interest in terms of stock, equity, or other financial interest in the sponsor company. In the United States the sponsor must also inform the FDA if the investigator owns more than $50,000 (Financial Disclosure by Clinical Investigators, 2008) of stock in a publicly traded company related to the drug under study. The National Institutes of Health, Office of Biotechnology Activities (2009) has issued a very helpful guideline about the informed consent process for gene transfer research, which contains helpful information and guidance about financial conflicts of interest for gene transfer research.

In recent years there has been concern about the extent to which the institution in which the clinical research takes place (e.g., a hospital or clinic) may have a conflict of interest. Hospitals and other investigative institutions may themselves act as sponsors, own patents and intellectual property, or be pursuing development programs by creating companies that may ultimately commercialize the drugs under development.

These activities can create financial conflict of interest situations. They must therefore ensure that they mitigate against any potential to not put patient interest first with appropriate procedures and checks and balances.

If you become aware that such conflicts exist, consider raising the matter with the PI and take your concerns to the EC, if necessary, for clarification. If you are uncomfortable with the situation and are unable to secure the necessary changes in the arrangements, it is best to avoid participation in such a clinical trial. A patient advocate may be able to help you work through the issues that arise in these situations.

Major regulatory authorities have their own good clinical practice auditors who visit clinical sites at the end of the program of clinical research to audit some of the investigative sites that took part in the clinical trials submitted in the marketing application. The purpose of these audits is to check the integrity of the clinical research process. The auditors check the clinical data that have been gathered to make sure that they are consistent with the data submitted in the marketing applications by the sponsors. Conflict of interest situations may be highlighted for investigative site audits. If financial conflicts of interest exist for certain investigators, their data may not be considered in the marketing application. This might mean that the drug under study cannot be approved for marketing.

Will the Investigator Be Too Busy to Take Care of Me during the Study?

You should ask how many other studies the clinical investigators are currently involved with to get an idea of how busy they are. Many PIs travel extensively to speak at conferences. You should ask which investigator will be overseeing your care when the PI is not available due to travel absences. If the clinical investigators are too busy to see you after you have enrolled in the clinical trial, you should view this as a red flag and thus a cause for concern. In this situation, you should bring this matter to the attention of the EC.

Your general practitioner is an excellent resource as you work through the issues of selecting a clinical trial. The following are some questions that may help you to start a conversation about clinical trials with the general practitioners and investigators concerned with your care.

Questions to Ask Your General Practitioner

1. Are you aware of any clinical trials that would be appropriate for my illness?
2. Are you aware of any reasons why I should not enroll in this clinical trial that I have identified?
3. Am I a suitable candidate for this clinical trial?

Questions to Ask the Principal Investigator before You Enroll in the Clinical Trial

General Questions to Consider Asking the Principal Investigator

1. Have you ever been barred from carrying out clinical research by any regulatory authority?
2. Have you ever been restricted in your ability to practice medicine?
3. Is this the best study for me?
4. If I participate in this clinical trial, will I be delaying the chance of receiving treatment with an already marketed drug? If so, what are the potential consequences for my health?
5. If I participate in this clinical trial, will I be damaging my prospects of being treated with currently available treatment?

6. Is this the best clinical trial for me at this point in the progress of my disease?

7. Is there a better alternative to this clinical trial for my specific situation?

8. Is there a potential benefit to me from participating in this clinical trial?

9. Does this clinical trial involve an experimental approach?

10. Does the study involve unacceptable risks for someone with my medical history? If so, what are the risks?

11. Is there sufficient understanding of this therapeutic approach for me to truly give my informed consent?

12. What is the Phase of study (Phase 1, 2, 3, or 4)?

13. What documentation or information regarding the medicines that I am currently taking, and have taken in the past do you want me to bring to my next meeting with you?

14. What documentation or information regarding my current illness, and previous medical history, do you want me to bring to my next meeting with you?

15. Are there any rules or safeguards built into the clinical trial to ensure that the risks are controlled and that I would be removed from the study if the drug was endangering my health?

16. What should I do if I experience a serious adverse event after enrolling in the clinical trial?

Questions to Help You to Determine if the Principal Investigator Has a Financial Conflict of Interest

1. Who is funding this study?

2. Do you have any ownership interest in the investigational agent that will be studied in the clinical trial?

3. Do you own stock in the company that is sponsoring this study?

4. Are you personally receiving payments for enrolling research subjects in this study?

5. Do you have a financial interest in the sponsor of this clinical trial?

Notes

1. Similar mechanisms may exist in other countries for physicians to sponsor clinical research.

2. Other similar requirements may exist in other countries, but the principles apply regardless of whether formal requirements are put in place by a regulatory authority.

References

Financial Disclosure by Clinical Investigators. (2008). 1 C. F. R. Title 21, Part 54.

National Institutes of Health, Office of Biotechnology Activities. (2003). *NIH Guidance on Informed Consent for Gene Transfer Research*. Retrieved January 29, 2010, from http://oba.od.nih.gov/oba/rac/ic/index.html

U.S. Department of Health and Human Services, Food and Drug Administration, Center for Drug Evaluation and Research (CDER), Center for Biologics Evaluation and Research (CBER), Center for Devices and Radiological Health (CDRH). (2001). *FDA Guidance Financial Disclosure by Clinical Investigators*. Silver Spring, MD: U.S. Department of Health and Human Services.

http://www.fda.gov/RegulatoryInformation/Guidances/ucm126832.htm

The Drug Development Process

Drug development is the process of moving a drug through animal and human testing, and registration to make it suitable for commercialization. This testing is required by international guidelines and regulations before a new medicine can be sold.[1] During the drug development process, researchers and regulatory authorities determine if the drug may be able to treat the disease that is being studied. During the process, researchers also determine if the drug will be safe. Because drug development is a complex process, we will spend sometime in this chapter exploring it; however, we will only be scratching the surface of what there is to know about the subject. If you are interested in finding out more, we suggest that you conduct a search on the Internet, using "drug development" as the search term. You can also find more information on this subject with the help of the librarian at your local library.

The Timeline and Cost for Drug Development

A new chemical entity (NCE) is a drug that is not approved for sale or that has been newly created in the laboratory. The process of drug development to find out if the NCE is safe and effective in humans can take 12 to 15 years or more. Drug development involves many organizations and individuals, such as hospitals, physicians, nurses, research subjects, health authorities, pharmaceutical companies/sponsors, clinical research organizations, and organizations that carry out toxicology studies in animals known as contract toxicology houses.

Novel medicines can cost over $800 million to develop (Adams & Brantner, 2006; DiMasi, Hansen, & Grabowski, 2003). This large sum of money includes the cost of failed development programs that were terminated. Although all aspects of drug development are expensive, clinical trial testing consumes most of a drug development budget.

Investors, venture capital firms (VCs), banks, and stockholders provide the money to fund drug development. Stakeholders and investors invest in the hope that if a drug is shown to be safe and effective, they will be paid back more than they invested after the drug is commercialized. Some sponsor companies receive funding from the federal government in the form of grants from the National Institutes of Health.

As mentioned above, although many drugs enter drug development, the number that is successfully registered and marketed is relatively small. The process of failure in development is known as attrition. The cost of drug development increases as the drug moves from preclinical to Phase 1, from Phase 1 to Phase 2, and from Phase 2 to Phase 3. Recent data suggest that approximately 62% of drugs taken into Phase 2 undergo attrition (Kola & Landis, 2004). Approximately 23% of drugs that enter the registration phase will fail to be approved. The overall success rate is approximately 11%.

Besides the number of drugs that are terminated during development and the registration process, a large number of drugs are abandoned every year for other reasons, some of them business related. It is difficult to quantify the number because this information is confidential to the individual companies. Drugs may be abandoned for any number of reasons—for safety problems or because the drug discovered does not have advantages over compounds already on the market or in development by competitors.

Drug Development Stages

As can be seen from Table 8.1 and Figure 8.1, drug development is divided into stages and is carried out in a stepwise way. This stepwise approach enables the sponsor company and the health authorities to determine if the drug is safe and effective enough to progress to the

Table 8.1 The Stages of Drug Development

The Stages of Drug Development	What Happens at Each Stage
Basic research	Knowledge is gained about the disease by studying the disease process and how it interacts with different drugs.
Drug discovery	This is the process that is used to discover new treatments.
Nonclinical development	This stage involves administering the drug to animals at high doses to find out how safe it might be when administered to patients.
Clinical research	This stage is divided into four phases: Phase 1, Phase 2, Phase 3, and Phase 4.
Drug registration	This is the process by which the drug is registered with different regulatory authorities around the world.
Commercialization	After registration by a regulatory authority, a drug can be commercialized in the country concerned. It can only be sold under the terms (known as a product label) authorized by the regulatory authority in the country concerned.

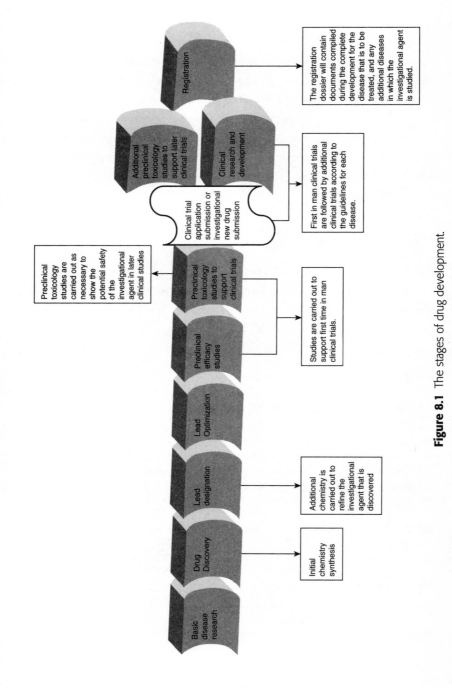

Figure 8.1 The stages of drug development.

next stage of drug development. A stepwise approach is important because the number of research subjects exposed at each phase usually increases, therefore increasing the potential for more research subjects to be harmed or to not experience benefit. At any point in the process it may be necessary to terminate a drug's development due to lack of effect or because it is unsafe.

Drug development begins with basic research that creates an understanding of the disease, its cause, and how it might be treated. Sometimes this research has been documented by other research groups, universities, and specialist organizations in published scientific papers. At other times it is carried out by pharmaceutical and biotechnology companies.

After basic research, the next step in the process is drug discovery. As the name implies, new medicines are discovered during this phase and can be found in different ways. They can be extracted from natural plants and herbs, or they can be designed synthetically on the basis of what is known about the causes of the disease. Drug discovery involves many different scientific disciplines, such as chemistry, biology, physiology, statistics, biochemistry, and biotechnology. During early drug discovery, drug testing may involve in vitro screens. During later stages of drug discovery, drugs are tested in whole animals, such as mice and rats. Animals can be bred to have diseases that are equivalent to those experienced by humans. The drug can be given to the "diseased" animals to see if the disease is treated effectively or eradicated. The dose that is needed to bring about an effect will be identified at this stage. By carrying out mathematical calculations, it is possible to estimate the dose that would be appropriate for administration to research subjects.

Many different types of studies are carried out in the laboratory during drug discovery and later during animal testing. One important type of study carried out in the laboratory is pharmacology studies. Pharmacology involves studying how the drug interacts with the diseased part of the body. Pharmacology studies are carried out in whole animals such as mice, rats, or on parts of animals to determine how a medicine works. For example, for a drug that is being developed to treat cardiovascular disease, pharmacology studies may involve studying the effect of the drug on the muscle of the heart, as well the effect on the whole body of mice and rats.

After demonstrating that a drug is efficacious against a disease in animal experiments, a new drug must be characterized.

Characterizing the Drug

During drug development it is important to fully understand the drug. The process by which knowledge is accumulated about the drug is known as characterization. The process of characterization involves learning as much about the drug as possible from a chemical point of view. For instance, it is important to know how easy it is to dissolve the drug in water. This is an example of a property of a drug that could impact how well it is able to treat the disease that is being studied. The level of acidity is an example of another property for which scientists will test the drug. After the drug is adequately characterized, the toxicology studies will be carried out to determine how safe the drug is in animals.

Toxicology Studies

Toxicology studies are carried out in animals and involve the administration of a drug to animals at higher doses than are given to research subjects. Sponsors only carry out tests that are required by regulatory authorities. These tests and studies are strictly regulated with the welfare of the animals in mind. Although great strides have been made to reduce animal testing, it is not possible to eliminate such testing altogether.

Major regulatory authorities such as the Food and Drug Administration (FDA, United States), the European Medicines Agency (EMEA, European Union), and the Ministry of Health and Welfare (MHW, Japan) collaborate with the International Conference of Harmonization (ICH) to develop guidelines on the toxicology studies to be carried out to support clinical trials. For instance, before studying a drug in women of childbearing age, it is necessary to carry out teratogenicity studies that evaluate if the drug will cause malformations in the offspring of the animals studied. These studies help sponsors to determine if a drug has the potential to damage the human fetus.

Toxicology guidelines provide an overview of how the toxicology studies should be designed and carried out. These guidelines provide sponsors with basic information, such as how many animals should be included in the toxicology studies, the species to be studied, and the doses to be given to the animals. The sponsors must then design their specific studies with the general guidelines in mind; because each drug is different, the exact designs will be dependent on the drug and the disease that is being studied. The duration of the toxicology studies will be dependent on the proposed duration of the clinical trials to be carried out. The duration of the clinical trials is dependent on the stage of the clinical program (Phase 1, 2, 3 or 4, and the type of disease that is being studied).

Table 8.2 Minimum Duration of Toxicology Studies to Support Clinical Trials*

Maximum Duration of Clinical Trial	Minimum Duration of Repeated Dose Toxicity Studies to Support Clinical Trials	
	Rodents	**Nonrodents**
Up to 2 weeks	2 weeks	2 weeks
Between 2 weeks and 6 months	Same as clinical trial	Same as clinical trial
>6 months	6 months	Up to 9 months, depending on the drug

* Reference: International Conference of Harmonization Tripartite Guideline, 1998.

Table 8.2 provides a summary of the duration of toxicology studies to be carried out in relation to the duration of the clinical trials (International Conference on Harmonization Tripartite Guideline, 1998). Toxicology studies will usually be carried out in one rodent and one nonrodent species unless it is clear that a second species is not needed after an appropriate amount of testing has been conducted (International Conference on Harmonization Draft Consensus Guideline, 2009). Testing in more than one species helps to identify when an effect that is seen is not relevant or is unlikely to happen in humans. Findings in animals that are not relevant for humans are called species-specific responses.

Toxicology studies intended to support the testing of a drug in research subjects (Table 8.3) must be carried out to good laboratory practice (GLP) standards. These are a set of international standards that ensure that toxicology studies provide meaningful results. Toxicology studies are divided into stages.

If the toxicology studies show that the drug is relatively safe, the drug can then be studied in clinical trials. Safety is a relative concept because it is defined in relation to the research subject's health status. For instance, a drug that might be considered relatively safe for a patient with cancer may be unsafe for a patient with a cold. After the toxicology studies are completed, and the health authority has given approval to start the clinical trial, it may commence (Chapter 3).

What Is Clinical Research?

After the toxicology studies are completed to the point to allow the clinical trials to start, the drug enters clinical research, if the process by which the drug is studied in research subjects. During clinical trials the drug's effect will be carefully documented. At the end of the study the results will be analyzed to determine if the drug is effective and safe. Clinical research makes it possible to determine the extent to

Table 8.3 Summary of Toxicology Studies

Type of Toxicology Study	Description
Acute toxicology studies	Acute toxicology studies determine toxic findings after single or short-term exposure to a chemical or drug in animals. Acute toxic effects usually occur within 14 days after administration of the chemical or drug. The chemical or drug is usually administered to the animal at much higher doses than will be administered during chronic toxicology studies.
Sub-acute toxicology studies	Sub-acute toxicology studies involve the repeated administration of a chemical or drug to animals at lower levels than were administered during acute toxicology studies. These studies involve the repeated administration of the drug for up to 90 days.
Chronic toxicology studies	Chronic toxicology studies involve the repeated administration of a chemical or drug to animals for longer periods of time to reproduce the real-life situation in humans. The period of time during which the chemical or drug is administered may last up to 12 months depending on the chemical or drug.
Carcinogenicity studies	Carcinogenicity studies involve the administration of a chemical or drug for 24 months, according to strict protocols agreed with the health authority, to determine if the chemical or drug may have a tendency to cause cancer in human beings.
Mutagenicity studies	Mutagenicity studies have the goal of determining if a chemical or drug is able to produce changes in cells that may predict a tendency to cause cancer.
Reproductive toxicology studies	Reproductive toxicology studies are designed to mimic the various stages of reproduction. The impact of a chemical or drug on fertility, formation of a fetus, and the postnatal stage after birth, including breast feeding, are studied in specially designed studies divided into three segments (Segment I, Segment II, and Segment III).
Juvenile toxicology studies	Juvenile toxicology studies are specially designed studies carried out on young animals to determine whether the chemical or drug impacts the development of the young animal. These studies provide helpful results to indicate risks before studies are carried out in young children and neonates.

which the drug has efficacy in a disease and how safe it might be if commercialized for use in the general patient population.

Although the design of the clinical trials will vary depending on the disease that the drug is being designed to treat, the clinical research will usually start out with studies that have the intention of finding an appropriate dose. The dose levels that will be administered to research subjects will be dependent on the drug and the disease. For instance, if testing a drug for pain relief, the doses that will be studied to find the best dose may be very low depending on how strong the pain relief is observed to be. If the pain relief provided by the drug is observed not to be very strong, higher doses will gradually be administered to see at what point pain relief is experienced.

Some of the initial studies will involve administration of the drug to healthy volunteers. The amount of drug in the bloodstream will be determined using tests that detect the levels at different times. These studies are known as pharmacokinetic studies.[2] During these studies, the goal is to determine what action the drug has on the body and also how the body handles the drug. Before a drug can exert a pharmacological effect on the human body, it will usually be absorbed into the bloodstream. After absorption, a drug will be distributed into the tissues and organs depending on how the drug has been designed and where it is intended to exert its pharmacological activity. The drug will begin to be broken down by a process of metabolism after administration or ingestion. Many drugs are broken down in the liver to produce metabolites. These metabolites may be pharmacologically active or inactive. After the metabolites are produced, they may remain in the body for a time depending on their half-lives before they are excreted by the process of elimination. The routes of elimination are the kidneys, the bile, and the lungs. If these routes of elimination are not working well, the drug and metabolites may build up in the body and cause adverse effects.

During drug development it is also important to determine how long the drug remains in the body and the time that it takes for 50% of the drug to be removed from the bloodstream, also known as the half-life of the drug. These factors influence how the drug acts when it is administered to a research subject. They may also impact if the drug will interact with other drugs that are being administered to the research subject.

The rates of absorption, distribution, metabolism, and elimination influence the amount of drug that should be administered to a research subject and therefore the determination of a dose at which the drug may be effective. Following the determination of appropriate dose(s), the next step in clinical research is to determine if efficacy occurs at the selected doses. During Phase 2, studies will be designed to find the best patient groups in which the drug works before advancing to larger scale Phase 3 studies to confirm that the drug works in larger groups of patients that are representative of real life.

Clinical Trial Monitoring

The process of overseeing the clinical trial is known as clinical trial monitoring. Clinical trial monitors work on behalf of the study sponsor and visit the investigative site every few weeks to review the clinical trial documentation. Monitoring helps to ensure that the protocol is adequately understood and adhered to by those involved with running the study. It can also help to identify if the principal investigator (PI) is not adequately protecting the rights of the research subjects. In other words, the study is also monitored to ensure that it conforms to good clinical practice (GCP; see Chapter 4). During the clinical trial, results for each research subject collected in the case report form are checked every few weeks to ensure that the information is being documented correctly by the study staff. Some of the CRFs may be reviewed at each visit for entry into a central study database. These results will be analyzed at the end of the study.

The Manufacturing Process

Materials to be given to research subjects in a clinical trial must be manufactured to very high standards. These standards are known as good manufacturing practice (GMP). Good manufacturing practice is a set of international standards established by regulatory authorities that must be adhered to by the international pharmaceutical industry during manufacturing. This standard helps to ensure that the material that is manufactured is free from contamination and is manufactured reproducibly and consistently. The pure drug in the medicine is what produces the drug activity. This is known as the active pharmaceutical ingredient (API). The complete medicine in the form of an injection, tablet, or syrup that contains the API is known as the formulation or drug product. You may see these terms in the informed consent document.

Role of Biotechnology and Molecular Biological Research

Biotechnology involves the use of living organisms such as bacteria, yeast, or enzymes to manufacture drugs and related products. Many breakthroughs in the treatment of hitherto untreatable disease have occurred with medicines made using biotechnology.

Scientists use genetic engineering and molecular biological techniques to increase their knowledge of how the human body works and how drugs may interact with the body to treat disease. Pharmaceutical companies use these techniques to efficiently screen which research subjects are likely to receive benefit from a specific drug. These techniques allow a better understanding of diseases and therefore the discovery of new potential targets or ways of treating disease. For instance, the understanding of genes and how they relate to disease is leading to the development of gene therapies (Chapter 9).

Patents

Patents are used by originators of drugs, processes, or devices to protect their inventions. They are very important to pharmaceutical companies to ensure that they can recuperate their investments. Patents provide for a term of protection from filing during which the originator has reserved the exclusive right to market the particular formulation without competition (e.g., 20 years in the United States). While many widget developers may only need to use a year of that time to develop their products, the amount of time used to develop drugs is often 10 to 12 years or longer, leaving a relatively short amount of time for commercial returns. Different regions of the world have instituted mechanisms for patent term restoration to add time back to the patent for time lost during the process of development and review.[3] With competition from generic manufacturers and the relatively high attrition rate for pharmaceutical drug development, the financial risks to pharmaceutical originators are significant.

Process of Drug Registration

The goal of carrying out studies during drug development is to secure registration to allow the drug to be sold to patients with the disease. Once a drug has successfully been studied in a series of preclinical (efficacy and toxicology), and clinical studies, all the data are gathered and submitted to the health authorities for approval. The health authority will review the information presented in the application to see if the drug is safe and effective in the patient population for which it is intended. The manufacturing site and the clinical investigative sites will be audited to make sure that the sponsor has carried out the research and development to the required standards.

During an audit at an investigative site, the health authority's inspector will visit the clinic or hospital. The inspector will make clear that he or she is on site to conduct an inspection and will ask for the documents that pertain to the clinical program that has been conducted by the sponsor. The inspector will review the data collected during the clinical trial and compare it to the data reported in the application that is under review by the health authority. The inspector will ensure that real patients were entered into the clinical trial and that the data in the regulatory submission match the data collected at the investigative site. If there are any discrepancies, the inspector will bring them to the attention of the reviewers at the health authority. The inspectors are specially trained to detect signs of fraud, such as the fabrication of results. The sponsor must have a successful inspection in order to be granted an approval. The inspection will usually last several days.

The GMP inspector will visit the manufacturing site(s) where the drug is manufactured and will conduct an inspection of the facility, reviewing the documentation collected during the years of development as well as analytical methods to ensure that these have been documented appropriately. If there are discrepancies between the data available at the manufacturing site and the data documented in the application that is under review, the application may not be approved. Each inspection may last several days.

The application assessment time varies from country to country. Drugs that have the potential to treat rare or serious unmet medical needs may be reviewed in a shorter time than other drugs in some countries. In the United States, drugs intended for unmet medical needs may be reviewed within 6 months (priority review). It usually takes at least 12 months for most drugs to be assessed to determine if they should be approved. The health authority will often ask questions and may require that additional studies are carried out before the application can be approved. If there are concerns about safety or if the drug does not appear to have sufficient efficacy according to the clinical trials carried out, the health authority may decide not to approve it and effectively issue a rejection.

During the approval process, the health authority will review all the data collected during drug development. If the drug is demonstrated by the sponsor to be safe, effective, and of good quality, the drug will be approved. The details of studies conducted and the results obtained will be described in the product label. The product label details the statements that a company can make about its product. The product label will detail the results of the animal and human studies. Most companies will file similar applications to many health authorities around the world seeking approval, so that the product can be marketed in as many countries as possible.

To illustrate some fictional examples of drug development programs, we will look at the programs of three companies: Oncomedicine, Arthrimed, and Rarimeds. Please note that all names are fictional and not intended to represent real-life companies or situations.

Oncomedicine Develops a Treatment for Head and Neck Cancer

Oncomedicine has developed Drug A for the treatment of head and neck cancer. Drug A was discovered in the laboratory by a university and was licensed in by Oncomedicine. Drug A had been protected extensively by patents by the university, and Oncomedicine has filed a number of additional patents throughout the world. Drug A underwent extensive drug discovery evaluations to see what produced the drug's anticancer activity. After this, Drug A was studied in several different animal models, which involved the testing of Drug A in mice with implanted tumors. Mice given Drug A were found to live longer than those given a placebo. These mice were also observed to no longer have tumors within several days of the administration. The toxicology program was carried out to good laboratory practice and was designed to closely mimic the intended use of Drug A in cancer patients. The toxicology studies also ensured that animals would receive about 30 times the dose that would be given to patients. The next step was to submit the Investigational New Drug application (IND) in order to conduct a clinical trial in the United States to see if the drug was as safe in humans as in animals. The IND summarized all animal work carried out to that point. It also explained how the drug would be made. Several clinical trial applications were submitted in several European countries after the IND was cleared for the first study to support the later clinical program.

In the first clinical trial, Drug A was administered to 25 research subjects with head and neck cancer to find a suitable dose. This first clinical trial involved injecting the drug into the tumor(s) and observing the responses. Patients remained in the hospital for 3 days after each injection for observation. Research subjects were administered one injection per week for 3 months. If the first dose level did not produce severe responses, the dose was increased and another group of patients was administered the drug. The responses from each different dose group were then compared. Additional dose finding studies were carried out in an additional 100 research subjects to assure that the dose results were reproducible. Later clinical trials involved careful measurements of tumor size. Because tumor size was seen to reduce at the higher doses, the higher dose was selected for the later Phase 2 and Phase 3 studies. After studying Drug A in 200 patients with head and neck cancer, eventually two Phase 3 studies were carried out that involved comparison with a drug already marketed for the treatment of head and neck cancer. The results showed that Drug A had a better survival than the drug already registered by 4 months. The drug application was prepared and submitted to the FDA, the EMEA (in Europe), and to the MHW (in Japan). Submissions will be made to regulatory authorities in other countries within the coming months. The health authorities will take between 6 months to 18 months, depending on the health authority, to approve the applications. After approval, the company can place the drug on the market in the countries in which it is approved.

If Drug A is not approved by any health authority, Oncomedicine will seek to address concerns, perhaps by carrying out additional clinical trials or by presenting the data in the application in different ways than they were originally presented in the application.

Arthrimed Develops a Treatment for Severe Rheumatoid Arthritis

Arthrimed has developed Drug B for severe rheumatoid arthritis. Drug B has been developed for patients in whom the currently available treatments are not effective or are not safe. Drug B was developed by Arthrimed and has taken 10 years from the time of first discovery to submission of the marketing authorization to the main regulatory authorities. The company has spent $650 million on the development. This figure does not include the failed drug programs for the same disease that have been terminated by Arthrimed due to safety and other problems.

Drug B had been protected extensively by patents by the company. Drug B underwent extensive drug discovery evaluations to see what produced the drug's anti-rheumatoid activity. The drug has been studied in several animal models to show that it is effective in healing arthritic lesions and reducing signs of pain. The toxicology studies made clear that patients with liver damage should not be administered Drug B.

The next step was to submit the IND to the FDA in order to conduct a clinical trial in the United States. Clinical trial applications were submitted to other countries to support the clinical program. The first clinical trial was carried out in healthy volunteers (Phase 1) and involved administering very low doses. Each research subject was observed for several days. Phase 2 clinical trials in patients with arthritis helped Arthrimed to determine the best doses for the Phase 3 program. Three large Phase 3 studies were conducted in 6000 patients in Europe, China, India, and Russia. These studies involved comparison of patients with severe arthritis on Arthrimed's drug and the already marketed treatment. The results showed that the patients on Arthrimed's drug had a better response than the patients on the available treatment. There were improvements in biological measures of inflammation and improvement in quality of life.

The drug application was prepared and submitted to the FDA, the EMEA (in Europe), and the MHW (in Japan). Submissions will be made to regulatory authorities in other countries within the coming months. The health authorities will take between 12 to 18 months, depending on the health authority, to approve the applications. After approval, the company will be able to place the drug on the market in the countries in which it is approved.

Rarimeds Develops Drug for Rare Genetic Disorder

Rarimeds has developed a treatment for a rare genetic disorder that affects 4000 people worldwide. The disease is caused by a protein that is not present in people affected by the disease. After demonstrating the efficacy of the drug in animal efficacy experiments, toxicology studies were carried out. These showed that the drug had a good safety profile. The clinical trials were carried out after the IND (USA) and clinical trial applications (other countries) were cleared. In the complete clinical program there were only 100 patients involved because of the rarity of the disease (30 in Phase 1, 20 in Phase 2, and 50 in Phase 3). Many countries around the world were involved in the clinical program. Many specialist investigative sites in each country that treat patients with the disease were involved in the clinical trial. Research subjects were studied for 12 months in each study. A number of research subjects showed reduction in the disease symptoms and a reduced need for other treatments. A laboratory test was also developed by Rarimeds to show patients who would benefit from Drug C.

At the end of the clinical program the authorization to market the drug was filed to all major health authorities. The drug is expected to be authorized within 6 months in most countries and within 12 months in others.

Notes

1. Major health authorities issue guidelines on the different aspects of drug development. The International Conference on Harmonization (ICH) issues guidelines that are used by companies to guide their drug development programs in addition to those issued by their national regulatory authorities.

2. Absorption, distribution, metabolism, and excretion (ADME) is used to describe the way that the human body handles a drug after it is administered.

3. In the United States in 1984, Waxman Hatch legislation gave 5 years of patent term restoration; Japanese legislation in 1988 gave up to 5 years restoration; in Europe, the supplementary protection certificate (SPC) allows for patent term restoration of up to 5 years.

References

Adams, C., & Brantner, V. (2006). Estimating the cost of drug development: Is it really 802 million dollars? *Health Affairs (Millwood)*, *25*(2), 420–428.

DiMasi, J., Hansen, R., & Grabowski, H. (2003). The price of innovation: New estimates of drug development costs. *Journal of Health Economics*, *22*(2),151–185.

International Conference on Harmonization Tripartite Guideline. (1998, September). *Duration of chronic toxicity testing in animals (rodent and non rodent toxicity testing)*. Available at http://www.ich.org/LOB/media/MEDIA497.pdf retrieved at January 29, 2010.

International Conference of Harmonization Draft Consensus Guideline (2009, October 29) Addendum to ICH S6: Preclinical Safety Evaluation of Biotechnology-Derived Pharmaceuticals (S6 R1). http://www.ich.org/LOB/media/MEDIA5784.pdf

Kola, L., & Landis, J. (2004). Can the pharmaceutical industry reduce attrition rates? *Nature Reviews*, *3*, 711–715.

Gene Transfer Clinical Research and Other Experimental Approaches

Tremendous advances are being made in the medical field every day. Novel approaches and molecular biological techniques are helping to address unmet medical needs by creating new approaches to treating disease. Some of these novel approaches are, nevertheless, experimental. An experimental drug is one that has not been fully evaluated in terms of its potential to treat disease or to do so safely.

Some examples of experimental approaches are cellular therapy, gene transfer also referred to as gene therapy, xenotransplantation (the transplantation of animal organs into the human body), stem cell approaches, and any approach that is unproven to cure or treat disease. Approaches involving vaccines, devices, tissues, or blood may also be experimental depending on the novelty of the approach. In addition, any drug that is being studied for the first time in Phase 1 (first-in-man studies) and early Phase 2 studies for novel drugs should be regarded as experimental. Some Phase 3 studies may need to be regarded as experimental, depending on how much data regarding the effectiveness of the approach are available. If these data are limited, you should regard the approach as experimental.

Some research subjects may be faced with a decision about whether to take part in studies that evaluate experimental drugs. Bear in mind that while such studies may be at the cutting edge of clinical research, they are nevertheless usually unproven. Because experimental drugs have not been demonstrated to be effective, descriptions of them in the informed consent document should avoid the use of misleading terms such as *treatment*, *therapy*, and *cure*. With experimental drugs the potential for such an agent to provide benefit is usually uncertain, and these terms can give research subjects false hope.

What Is an Unmet Medical Need?

Many experimental drugs are studied in patients who have serious life-threatening illnesses. These are often referred to as unmet medical needs. An unmet medical need is a disease or condition that is not addressed adequately by currently available treatment. A few examples of diseases that are considered unmet medical needs are most if not all cancers, systemic lupus erythematosus, most if not all rare diseases, and Alzheimer disease. An understanding of biology and some understanding of molecular biology will help you to understand the terminology likely to be included in the informed consent document if you are considering taking part in a clinical trial involving an experimental drug or approach. We will explore biology briefly on the next few pages.

Cells: Building Blocks of the Human Body

Advances in molecular biology and biochemistry have enabled us to understand the cell and its components to a much greater extent than was previously possible. The human body is made up of trillions of cells

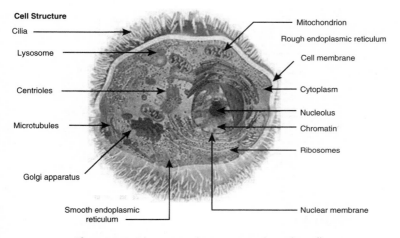

Figure 9.1 Diagrammatic representation of a cell.

(Fig. 9.1). These cells are too small to see with the naked eye, but they can be seen in great detail using a powerful microscope. Each cell fulfills a purpose in the body, according to its location and type, and is highly organized. Each cell contains organelles, or "mini-factories." Some examples of organelles are the nucleus, chromosomes, rough endoplasmic reticulum, the cell membrane, the nucleolus, centrioles, and ribosomes. The cell nucleus contains a set of chromosomes. Each chromosome contains deoxyribonucleic acid (DNA). DNA contains genes, which determine heritable characteristics, such as eye and hair color.

DNA

A DNA molecule consists of two strands that coil around to form a double helix which consists of base pairs. The four bases are adenine (A), thymine (T), guanine (G), and cytosine (C). Only A–T or T–A will pair together. Likewise, only G–C or C–G will pair together. The pairing causes DNA to form into a double helix (Fig. 9.2). The cell nucleus

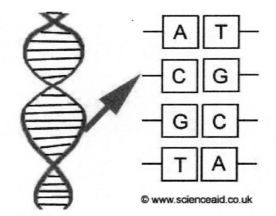

Figure 9.2 The DNA shown as a coil and when broken out into its base pairs.

contains the DNA and is the command center for the cell, in the same way that the brain is the command center for the human body.

Genes

One important component of DNA is the gene. Each cell in the human body contains about 25,000 to 35,000 genes. These days, people often talk about their genes. You have probably heard people say things like "It is in my genes" or "This disease has been in our family for centuries." Human genes are small pieces of code or information that are located on DNA. These pieces of code tell the body how to operate. Genes carry information that determines our physical traits, such as the color of our eyes, skin, and hair. The complete set of genes in an organism is known as its genome. An individual's genome will have an influence on their potential to develop certain diseases.

Many diseases are inherited. When this is the case, genes are involved. Defective genes can be transferred from one generation to another in the same way that hair color can be passed on from parent to child via genes that direct hair color. Some examples of inherited diseases are hemophilia, cystic fibrosis, and sickle cell anemia.

Diseases that are inherited sometimes involve a missing protein due to the presence or absence of a particular gene. Proteins direct many body processes and are produced in the cells by genes. When the message in the gene is not translated correctly in the cell, the correct protein may not be produced, and the patient may develop a disease as a result. By replacing the missing gene, the protein can be produced, and the disease may be cured or treated as a result. The genetic code is the set of rules by which information encoded in a gene is translated into a protein. The technique of replacing faulty genes can be used to produce the protein that the defective gene was unable to produce. Gene transfer is an example of an experimental approach that has had some remarkable successes (Cideciyan et al., 2009; Miller & Stamatoyannopoulos, 2001; Wartiovaara, 2000). We will spend some time reviewing gene transfer as an example of experimental approaches that you may come across.

Gene Transfer

Gene transfer is an experimental approach that involves the insertion of genes to correct a disease process. Such diseases that may be amenable to this approach are cystic fibrosis, hemophilia, sickle cell anemia, and severe combined immunodeficiency (SCID), to name only a few. The purpose of gene transfer is to correct the disease process that has resulted from a defective gene. Such illnesses or conditions may be caused by the absence of a needed protein or the presence of a defective protein. Gene transfer introduces the missing genes into the body to replace faulty or missing genes. By so doing, it is believed that it will be possible to treat or cure disease.

The eventual hope is that for some diseases, like hemophilia, the transferred genes will keep working throughout a person's lifetime. There may be gene transfer uses that would only require short-term gene activity, such as growth of new blood vessels or wound repair. Advances in human gene transfer may allow doctors to treat a disease or abnormal medical condition by turning off a faulty gene to stop the growth of a cancerous tumor, for example. Or they may allow the body to begin producing a necessary protein or other substance, such as an enzyme, that the faulty gene cannot direct the body to produce.

There have been some examples of success in the use of gene transfer approaches. Hemophilia is caused by the deficiencies in clotting factor VIII (FVIII) and factor IX (FIX). These factors are created in the liver and secreted into the blood, where they bring about the formation of blood clots when a person experiences a cut or other trauma and bleeds. Without these factors a person will bleed to death when injured. The use of gene transfer to transfer the genes responsible for the production of the genes that make the factors has had a measure of success in animal experiments and in human clinical trials (Miller & Stamatoyannopoulos, 2001).

All genes have regions that are responsible for overseeing protein production. Some terms that you may come across in the informed consent document are *promoters*, *introns*, and *operons*. Suffice it to say that these are parts of the gene that govern how it will act when inserted in the body. They will not be considered further in this book.

Different Types of Gene Therapy/Gene Transfer

To transfer a gene into the body, a method that can effectively introduce the gene must be used. There are viral and nonviral methods for introducing genes into cells to produce the required protein. The viral approach is believed to be able to make more protein than the nonviral approach.

The Regulatory Process for Gene Transfer

Gene transfer is a biological intervention, and therefore there are safeguards that must be built into the regulatory review to ensure research subject safety and well-being. Regulatory and other mechanisms for oversight for gene transfer research will vary from country to country. In the United States safeguards exist to ensure that there is adequate protection for research subjects and professional staff handling the material. In the United States the organizations that review gene transfer experiments are the Food and Drug Administration (FDA), the Institutional Review Board (IRB), the Institutional Biosafety Committee (IBC; see also Chapter 3), and the Recombinant DNA Advisory Committee (RAC). The RAC is a committee comprised of medical, scientific, ethical, and lay people. The meetings are held in public to allow public debate about this field of research. The IRB, IBC, FDA, and RAC work together to ensure that only the studies that meet the necessary requirements can commence in research subjects. The interrelationship of the various regulatory bodies in the United States that oversee gene transfer research is shown in Figure 9.3. Guidelines were first issued by the National Institutes of Health (NIH) in 1976. They have evolved as the field has evolved. An update was issued in 2002 (National Institutes of Health, 2002).

In other countries the mechanisms for review and approval of gene transfer research may vary from that in the United States, although the principles involved may be similar. For example, in the United Kingdom, the Gene Therapy Advisory Committee is responsible for the ethical oversight of all gene transfer research. Some countries may not have formal mechanisms for regulating gene transfer research or experimental approaches. Even in the latter situations, this chapter will

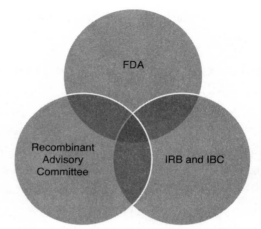

Figure 9.3 Organizations that are involved with the oversight of gene transfer clinical research in the United States.
Key: FDA–Food and Drug Administration; IRB–Institutional Review Board; IBC–Institutional Biosafety Committee.

help you to navigate the likely issues that you should be aware of in considering whether to enroll in an experimental clinical trial.

The Regulatory Process for Other Experimental Drugs and Approaches

The regulatory process for other experimental approaches such as cell therapies and stem cell therapies will vary depending on the type of experiment to be conducted in research subjects and the country in which the experimental clinical research is to be conducted. All clinical protocols for experimental approaches will undergo regulatory review by the health authority, as well as an ethics review by the ethics committee (EC). Additional reviews may be required by committees focused on safety, similar to the IBC in the United States.

Potential Safety Concerns with Gene Transfer and Experimental Approaches

There are a number of potential safety concerns with gene transfer. These concerns are greater with the viral approaches than with the nonviral approaches; they include allergic reactions, inflammation, and difficulty controlling the amount of protein produced. If you are involved with a viral gene transfer clinical trial, you may be asked to undergo safety evaluations during the clinical trial and after the clinical trial is completed, for several months, years, or even for the rest of your life. Your spouse or partner may also need to be evaluated. It is very important that you make every effort to attend the visits, where you will be carefully examined and evaluated. You should also report any side effects or adverse events that you experience during and after the clinical trial, even if you are unsure if they may be related to the gene transfer clinical research. This will enable researchers to gather as much information as possible about the safety of gene transfer research and help them to intervene if you are experiencing adverse events related to the gene transfer approach.

One theoretical concern with viral gene transfer involves integration of the virus into the genome to affect future generations. It is important to ensure that you have a good understanding of the theoretical as well as actual risks as you consider enrolling in an experimental clinical trial.

You may hear many stories of cures and be tempted to enroll in clinical trials or to purchase experimental therapies from countries with fewer regulatory hurdles than in your own country. It is important to remember that until controlled studies have been carried out by sponsors, any reports of cures and improvements must be regarded as anecdotal. They must be shown to have stemmed from the gene transfer or experimental approach in rigorously designed and conducted clinical trials. The true validation of an experimental approach is the grant of a marketing authorization by a major health authority.

Update on Progress Made with Gene Transfer Research

At the time of writing, there are no approved treatments for gene transfer, although some very promising results have been observed in clinical trials (Cideciyan et al., 2009; Miller & Stamatoyannopoulos, 2001; Wartiovaara, 2000). While gene transfer has tremendous promise, there have been a number of setbacks, some of them to do with safety, which have slowed the field down.

Stem Cell Clinical Research

There are two types of stem cells: adult stem cells and embryonic stem cells. If you have ethical issues with the use of embryonic stem cells, the adult stem cell approach may be more acceptable to you. There may be the potential for stem cell research to produce cures in the future. As a research subject, it is important to carefully review the findings from animal efficacy studies, as well as any safety concerns that have come to light from the toxicology studies conducted. There have been anecdotal reports of people experiencing improvements in their symptoms from stem cell approaches administered in clinics in different countries around the world. As encouraging as these reports are, until controlled clinical trials are carried out and reviewed by health authorities leading to a marketing authorization, the stem cell approach must be regarded as experimental. It is difficult to know the source of the improvement in symptoms outside of controlled clinical trials. There are diseases in which the symptoms are variable over time. Some diseases respond to the placebo effect—they seem to improve even if a placebo is administered. For these reasons, controlled clinical trials are important to demonstrate that any improvements or apparent cures were actually the result of administration of the stem cell or other experimental approaches.

Beware of False Promises

Patients who are seriously ill are often desperate for a cure. Have you ever been in a desperate situation that left you feeling vulnerable and open to suggestions? This also happens when a person is very unwell, in pain, or hoping for a final solution to a chronic illness. Remember that if it sounds too good to be true, it probably is. When faced with a serious illness, it is easy for one to put greater credence on experimental results than one should. Unfortunately, experimental approaches are sometimes the subject of hype. A patient advocate or someone acting in that role may be able to help you to sift through the available results. If data from controlled clinical trials are not available, then any results that are presented to you should be considered suspect. Jackie is an example of someone who was in a desperate situation.

Jackie's Story

Jackie was a terminally ill cancer patient. Her physician advised her that the only option for her going forward would be palliative treatments. He explained that these would help to maintain her quality of life, but he made it clear that they would not cure her underlying disease. She felt desperate. She needed to do something. She searched online and found a Phase 1 clinical trial at a university hospital in another part of the country involving an experimental approach. She made travel and hotel arrangements after speaking to the clinical trial coordinator, and she traveled to the hospital site later that week to meet with the principal investigator (PI). The PI was very optimistic about the clinical trial. He spoke enthusiastically about the results observed to that point of the clinical trial. He explained that the experimental drug had only been administered to three previous research subjects. Each of these three research subjects had received the first dose according to the clinical protocol. At least 10 additional doses were planned in the clinical trial. He explained to Jackie that if she agreed to enroll in the clinical trial, and if she met the inclusion/ exclusion criteria, she would be the first research subject to receive the second of 10 planned doses according to the clinical protocol. Jackie asked a lot of questions, but she felt under pressure to do something that might prolong her life.

Points to Consider

1. Jackie has terminal cancer. By not involving her general practitioner or specialist in her evaluation of this clinical trial, she is quite vulnerable to being persuaded to take part in this Phase 1 clinical trial.

2. She should have brought a relative or friend with her that could act as a patient advocate, or requested one from the investigative site, but she did not. She is therefore alone and has no one with whom to discuss what she has heard. She feels "pressured" to take part in the clinical trial, although the investigator has made it clear to her that the drug is unproven and experimental and that the Phase 1 clinical trial is the first dose finding study.

3. The investigator appears to be positive about the potential of the drug. Although he has made clear that it is a Phase 1 study, and the agent is experimental, his positive attitude, demeanor, and enthusiasm are misleading. This could give Jackie false hope that the drug will cure her disease.

4. This is a Phase 1 study, and the drug is in an early dose-finding study. This does not appear to be a clinical trial that will prolong Jackie's life. She is vulnerable and at risk of entering the study for the wrong reasons.

Questions to Ask If You Are Considering Entering a Study Involving an Experimental Approach or Drug

1. Will this clinical trial involve an experimental agent or approach, or biological agent?
   a. If so, what precautions are in place to ensure that side effects will be monitored during the clinical trial?
   b. If so, what precautions are in place to ensure that possible long-term side effects are monitored after the clinical trial is completed?
2. Were allergic reactions or antibody formation observed in the animal studies that might indicate the potential for allergic reactions during the clinical trial?
3. How many patients will be enrolled in the clinical trial?
4. How many other studies have already been carried out in this program?
5. Is there enough understanding of the science for me to be able to give informed consent to the proposed approach?
6. How long will I need to be monitored for adverse events and side effects after leaving the study?
7. Are there any theoretical or real concerns about future generations from my participation in this clinical trial?

References

Cideciyan, A. V., Hauswirth, W. W., Aleman, T. S., Kaushal, S., Schwartz, S. B., Boye, S. L., et al. (2009). Vision 1 year after gene therapy for Leber's congenital amaurosis. *New England Journal of Medicine, 361*(7), 725–727.

Miller, D. G., & Stamatoyannopoulos, G. (2001). Gene therapy for hemophilia. *New England Journal of Medicine, 344*, 1782–1784.

National Institutes of Health. (2002). *Guidelines for research involving recombinant DNA molecules.* Retrieved on December 30, 2009, from http://www.oba.od. nih.gov/rdna/nih_guidelines_oba.html

Wartiovaara, K. (2000). Gene therapy approaches to neurodegenerative disease. *Neural Notes, 5(3)*, 5–8.

Clinical Trials Involving the Elderly

In this chapter we will consider the role of the elderly in clinical trials. The elderly are patients above 65 years of age. They consume a large number of medicines, yet they are underrepresented in clinical trials (Bene, & Liston, 1997; Bugeja, Kumar, & Banerjee, 1997; Siu, 2007). This is unfortunate because the adverse event and side effect profile of a drug cannot be completely understood until it is adequately studied in the population in which it will be used. Consequently, the elderly are prone to experience unexpected adverse reactions and side effects not observed during clinical trials after a new drug is commercialized.

Why the Elderly Are Often Excluded from Clinical Trials

There are several reasons why the elderly may be excluded from clinical trials. To increase the chances of a drug's success, the sponsor formulates exclusion criteria that are designed to assure the relative good health of research subjects so that patients with serious health problems are largely excluded. Protocols are generally written to exclude research subjects who have liver and kidney function that are not optimal. This is because healthy livers and kidneys are needed to handle drugs administered during the clinical trial. The incidence of health problems increases with age, consequently elderly patients are often excluded from many clinical trials. To assure the health of research subjects, many trials have age cut-offs to exclude those above 65 years of age. There can be a reluctance to treat diseases such as cancer aggressively in the elderly. And, in some countries, the result of the aforementioned factors is that unless the disease is mostly present in the elderly, as a group, the elderly may not be included in large numbers in clinical trials. Consequently, the elderly are often excluded from studies that test novel drugs for diseases like cancer which afflict the elderly at a highrate.

During the later stages of drug development, population trials may be carried out by sponsors to determine how safe and effective the drug is in different populations, including the elderly, and research subjects with renal and liver dysfunction. Despite this, by the time a drug is registered, the elderly population exposed to the drug is often relatively small. Consequently, the real experience with a drug in the elderly is often gained after the drug is on the market. Doctors effectively have to try to find the best dose for the elderly in uncontrolled situations as a result of the deficiencies of the clinical trial process.

For diseases that occur primarily in the elderly, clinical trials will be carried out in the elderly. Alzheimer disease is an example of such a disease. When sponsors wish to include the elderly in clinical trials, there are challenges that must be acknowledged and managed. Let us consider Clint's story.

Clint's Story

Clint is a patient with early-onset Alzheimer disease. His son is his main caregiver and he has decided to place Clint in a clinical trial to test a new drug that is being studied in patients with early-onset Alzheimer disease. The purpose of the clinical trial is to test a liquid form of a drug that has already been registered as a tablet in several countries. The clinical trial will involve several hospital stays over an 8-week period.

Points to Consider

1. This type of clinical trial is attractive to those taking care of patients with Alzheimer disease because the medicine is documented as relatively safe and effective in a previously registered format, the tablet.
2. This type of clinical trial is conducted to demonstrate that a liquid formulation is not essentially different in the effects produced from the tablet formulation, which is already registered in several countries.
3. The weekend stays at the investigative site will provide respite for his son.
4. Clint will be given thorough medical checkups during the clinical trial, and he will be able to leave the clinical trial if he is adversely affected by the medicine.
5. As attractive as the potential for respite care is, Clint's son should ensure that this medication is the best treatment for his father at this point in his disease. If he is already effectively controlled on another medication, it would not be appropriate to remove this medication so that he can be enrolled in this clinical trial. However, this type of trial might be of benefit to Clint if he cannot swallow his current treatment provided in the form of tablets; a liquid formulation might be easier for him to ingest.

Finding Solutions to the Potential Challenges of Elderly Participation in Clinical Trials

Sponsors, the elderly, and their caregivers face a number of challenges as far as participation of the elderly in clinical trials is concerned. The following is a list of some challenges, but it is not comprehensive:

- As a result of compromised physiological systems, some elderly research subjects may be prone to a higher incidence of adverse events than younger research subjects.
- The elderly may not have easy access to information about clinical trials. For instance, they may not have access to or know how to use a computer; therefore, they may not be able to access the Internet.
- The elderly often suffer from several different diseases at the same time and therefore take several medications concomitantly. This can lead to the potential for interactions between these medications, as well as with the drug under study.
- The elderly are not always able to understand complicated clinical trial instructions or to use electronic patient diaries without support. This can reduce their compliance during clinical trials.
- The elderly may not have the support of relatives or friends to ensure that they can attend scheduled clinical trial visits. In these situations, the assistance of patient advocates will be vital to assure compliance during the clinical trial.
- The elderly may not be able to understand the information presented in the informed consent form. It can take more time and resources to make sure that they are adequately informed and consented.
- The elderly may be prone to unforeseen complications during the clinical trial, particularly if they are frail. For instance, the elderly take many medications, some of which may have a tendency to cause falls. These falls would be documented in the case report form (CRF)

as adverse events and could be linked to the drug, although they may be caused by other medications being taken concomitantly by the elderly research subject.

• The elderly must be monitored carefully during clinical trials. This may include the use of at-home visits by clinical trial staff.

As daunting as the above challenges are, none of them need be insurmountable. Each of these potential or real issues can be addressed, particularly if the elderly research subject needs to participate in a clinical trial because of his or her need to access novel or potentially effective therapies. The clinical trial staff can work with the sponsor and the elderly research subject to find solutions to many of these problems. The patient advocate can work with research subjects and their families to ensure that there is sufficient understanding of the information that is presented in the informed consent form before it is signed. The patient advocate can also organize support, perhaps in the form of a visiting nurse, to ensure that the elderly research subject is compliant with the study procedures.

What can you do if you or a relative is being excluded from a clinical trial on the basis of age or because of the challenges discussed above? You can contact the principal investigator (PI) and explore possible solutions. The PI can request permission from the sponsor to include the patient, provided the patient otherwise meets the inclusion and exclusion criteria. If an exemption cannot be made, the PI may be able to prescribe the drug on a compassionate basis.

Nowadays it is recognized that the physiological health of a research subject is as important as the chronological age. With people living longer and paying more attention to nutrition and exercise, the current attitude of arbitrary age cut-offs may need to be re-examined.

The number of patients that are considered elderly (65 years and over) is expected to double by the year 2030 (Yancik, 2005). The inclusion of elderly patients in clinical trials is therefore an issue that will need to be addressed by the pharmaceutical industry and regulators. In the meantime, discussion of these issues with the PI may lead to solutions on an individual basis. Regulatory authorities have issued guidances on this subject that you may wish to review (Committee for Human Medicinal Products, 2006; FDA Guideline for Industry, 1994; International Conference on Harmonization of Technical Requirements for Registration of Pharmaceuticals for Human Use, 1993; U. S. Department of Health and Human Services, 2001).

Questions to Ask the Principal Investigator and Study Staff If You Are Elderly or Caring for an Elderly Patient

1. Will I be provided with any devices to help me to remain compliant during the clinical trial?
2. Will I be able to meet with a patient advocate to help me to understand the clinical trial before signing the informed consent form?
3. As a caregiver of a research subject with Alzheimer disease, can someone be assigned to help me to follow the study procedures properly?

References

Bene, J., & Liston, R. (1997). The special problems of conducting clinical trials in elderly patients. *Reviews in Clinical Gerontology, 7*, 1–3.

Bugeja, G., Kumar, A., & Banerjee, A. K. (1997). Exclusion of elderly people from clinical research: A descriptive study of published reports. *British Medical Journal, 315*, 1059.

Committee for Human Medicinal Products, European Medicines Agency. (CHMP/ EMEA). (2006). *Adequacy of guidance on the elderly regarding medicinal products for human use*. EMEA/498920/2006. Retrieved December 31, 2009, from http://www.emea.europa.eu/pdfs/human/opiniongen/49892006en.pdf

FDA Guideline for Industry. (1994). *Studies in support of special populations: Geriatrics.* ICH-E7. August 1994.

International Conference on Harmonisation of Technical Requirements for Registration of Pharmaceuticals for Human Use. (1993, June). *ICH harmonised tripartite guideline studies in support of special populations: Geriatrics, E7, Step 4,* from http://www.ich.org/cache/compo/276-254-1.html

Siu, L. L. (2007). Clinical trials in the elderly – A concept comes of age. *New England Journal of Medicine, 356*(15), 1575–1576.

U. S. Department of Health and Human Services, Food and Drug Administration, Center for Drug Evaluation and Research (CDER), Center for Biologics Evaluation and Research (CBER). (2001). *Guidance for industry content and format for geriatric labeling.* Retrieved on December 30, 2009, from http://www.fda.gov/downloads/Drugs/GuidanceComplianceRegulatoryInformation/Guidances/ucm075062.pdf

Yancik, R. (2005). Population aging and cancer: A cross national concern. *Cancer Journal, 11*(6), 437–441.

Clinical Trials Involving Children

11

Historically, medicines have been administered to children in the absence of adequate clinical trial data. Many medicines studied only in adults are still being prescribed for and administered to children. There are a number of reasons for this. An important one is the ethical concern of conducting clinical trials in children. Children cannot understand complicated scientific information about drugs under study and experimental approaches. This makes it impossible to obtain informed consent from them. There are also logistical and practical challenges involved with carrying out clinical trials in children. Because of these and other challenges, sponsors have a tendency to put off conducting clinical trials in children, and they often never conduct trials, even after the drug is registered for many years for use in adults. Some of these challenges are explored in this chapter and suggestions are provided for how parents and guardians can work through them.

Ethical Concerns with the Conduct of Clinical Trials in Children

As explained in Chapter 4, informed consent must be given before a research subject can take part in a clinical trial. Legally, children are considered unable to give informed consent, and their parents or guardians are required to grant informed consent on their behalf. This raises other issues from an ethical point of view, particularly if children are required to undergo painful or uncomfortable procedures as part of a clinical trial. Children may refuse to take part because of anticipated or real discomfort. In accordance with the Declaration of Helsinki, children should not be forced to enter clinical trials against their will, even if there is a potential for benefit.

Balancing Risks with Benefits in Clinical Trials in Children

Because of the difficulties of obtaining informed consent from children, it is crucial to ensure that the potential benefits of the clinical trial are carefully balanced against the risks inherent in the clinical trial. The child should have the disease that is being studied and should have the potential to derive benefit from participation in the clinical trial. Parents who are considering whether to enroll their child in a clinical trial should be provided with the data obtained from preclinical and clinical studies already completed. This will enable them to gain an understanding of the risks, side effects, and adverse effects that came to light during those trials; this information should be explained thoroughly by the investigator. After the data have been evaluated, a judgment will need to be made by the parent or guardian regarding whether to enroll the child into the clinical trial. Gregory and Dana have faced many of these types of issues.

Gregory and Dana's Experience

Gregory and Dana are the parents of Derek, a 5-year-old child with a rare autoimmune disease that only occurs in children. Children suffering from this disease do not live to reach adulthood because of the resulting disease complications. Derek's condition is currently controlled by a marketed medicine, a corticosteroid, which has been able to treat the symptoms, but not cure the underlying disease. The long-term side effects of this treatment are expected to be significant. They have heard about an experimental gene therapy that is being investigated in a clinical trial in a local teaching hospital. They have read many claims in the local press suggesting that this might theoretically be a miracle cure for their son's disease. This would be the first Phase 1 study of the gene therapy approach in pediatric patients like their son. After much discussion, they are still struggling to make a decision.

Points to Consider

1. The study is a Phase 1 first-in-man study. It would seem prudent given Derek's medical situation not to enroll him in the clinical trial at this time but to reassess the decision after additional data from later phases of the clinical trial are available, perhaps in older children.

2. Their son is currently controlled on available medication. The possibility of Derek being able to continue taking the corticosteroid if he enters the clinical trial should be explored with the principal investigator (PI). Corticosteroids cannot be stopped abruptly, and therefore this is an important question.

3. In order to enable the PI to evaluate Derek for enrollment in the clinical trial, the parents must provide the PI with very thorough medical and medication histories during their discussions to ensure that any potential drug–drug interactions can be avoided. Their son is in fragile health; therefore, it is important not to do anything that would destabilize his medical condition.

4. Given that the gene therapy has not yet been evaluated in children, it is very likely that any results implying a miracle cure have come from studies in animals. These types of data can lead to hyped headlines in the major newspapers, so it is important that the data are researched and reviewed objectively by parents in these situations. Certainly, the gene therapy cannot be considered a miracle cure until adequately controlled studies are carried out in sufficient numbers of pediatric research subjects and the application for marketing authorization is approved by the health authority.

5. In diseases where data may exist from adult patients with the same disease, parents or guardians should ask the PI if any dose-finding studies have been carried out in teenagers or young adults with their son's illness. The results of these studies may enable them to determine the types of issues that might arise if they place their son in this study. However, it must be borne in mind that teenagers and young adults may be different from children 5 years and younger in terms of dosing and safety. Therefore, safety and dosing data from older children cannot simply be extrapolated to younger children.

6. A patient advocate can assist parents like Gregory and Dana in sifting through data so that they can make this difficult decision.

Logistical and Practical Difficulties of Conducting Clinical Trials in Children

Conducting clinical trials in children can cause more logistic and practical difficulties than the same or similar clinical trials in an adult population. For example, during clinical trials, research subjects must provide feedback on adverse events and side effects experienced during the clinical trial. Children may be unable to give intelligible feedback in this respect. This can be particularly difficult in very young children. To get around this challenge, parents and guardians must question children carefully as they go through the clinical trials to learn of any new sensations or discomforts. They should carefully examine their child after administration of a drug for new skin rashes and observe them for any changes in behavior or ailments, since these could be signs of adverse events. Sometimes clinical trials are not the best option for children, as we will see from Raymond and Brenda's story.

Raymond and Brenda's Story

Raymond and Brenda are parents of an emotionally disturbed child, Brian. They want to avoid putting him on medication, but they have begun to consider enrolling him in a clinical trial. The clinical trial will involve the comparison of drug therapy with cognitive-behavioral therapy. There is a 50% chance that their son will be randomized to drug therapy if they enroll him in this clinical trial.

Points to Consider

1. Since the parents are against the administration of drug therapy to their son, this clinical trial is not appropriate because there is a 50% chance that he will be randomized to drug therapy.
2. Raymond and Brenda would be well advised to identify a cognitive-behavioral therapist specializing in the treatment of children like their son. The therapist will be able to develop a program of treatment for their son outside of the constraints of a clinical trial. Alternatively, a clinical trial involving cognitive approaches to controlling behavior may also be an option.

Although placebos may be used in study designs involving children, the appropriateness of inclusion of placebos will depend on the therapeutic area. Children should not be exposed to placebos for long periods of time without adequate treatment. In some disease situations, placebo study designs will not be appropriate. For instance, in situations involving studies on anti-epileptic medication, appropriate study designs involving children may involve the addition of the new drug to already approved treatment to determine if the new drug produces a better effect when added to the currently approved drug. As this example illustrates, study designs should be adjusted to take into account the need to assure adequate treatment for certain diseases in studies involving children.

The Regulatory Environment for Pediatric Clinical Trials

Because companies have tended not to carry out clinical trials in children, many medicines are used in children in the absence of safety and efficacy data in this population. This is known as off-label use. Product labels will often state that there is no clinical trial experience in children or insufficient experience to provide very much guidance. Although physicians and others treating children with these medicines have gained experience in this population, this is not the ideal situation. The problem with this status quo is that the decision on how a child should be treated is left up to the treating physician or a hospital.

The implementation of legislation and guidelines has helped change this status quo, encouraging and requiring clinical trials in children in some situations. In addition, studies are required in children if the condition the drugs are being developed to treat occurs in the pediatric population. A sample of the available guidelines is provided at the end of this chapter under the References. Additional guidelines can be found at http://www.fda.gov and http://www.emea.eu. Companies are encouraged to conduct clinical trials in children, using incentives such as extended patent life or data exclusivity. By carrying out these clinical trials, companies can recuperate their development costs and have the potential to earn a profit. The United States has seen an increase in the number of clinical trials conducted in children as a result of these measures. Companies will need to obtain formal waivers if clinical trials are not to be carried out in children for medicines to be used in children after marketing in the United States and in Europe. The European Union's incentives in the form of marketing exclusivity and patent term extensions are similar to those available in the United States.

In Europe and the United States there are regulatory mechanisms in place to ensure that the protocol designs of studies to be conducted in children are thoroughly reviewed and commented upon before the study can be initiated. The ethics committees (ECs) at the investigative sites will also review the protocols.

Questions to Ask before Entering Your Child into a Clinical Trial

As a parent or guardian, your primary concern in entering your child in a clinical trial will be to ensure your child's safety and well-being during the trial. It is important to review the information presented to you about the clinical trial before giving your consent. On the following pages you will find some questions you can ask the PI about the suitability of a clinical trial for your child. In addition to the basic questions that should be asked about pediatric research subjects, additional questions should be raised if your child has a rare disease.

Questions to Ask before Entering Your Child into a Clinical Trial

1. How many adults or other children have already been exposed to this drug in the clinical trial setting?

2. What was the side effect profile that was observed in adults?

3. Were the side effects and adverse effects observed to occur in adults at any particular doses?

   a. If yes, how will these doses relate to the doses to be studied in my child?

   b. How will the blood levels of drug observed in adults relate to the expected blood levels anticipated in my child?

4. Who will pay for medical treatment if my child is injured during the clinical trial or suffers adverse events or side effects that require treatment?

5. Are there any rules or safeguards built into the clinical trial to ensure that the risks are controlled and that my child would be removed from the trial if safety becomes an issue?

6. Have any studies been conducted in juvenile animals?

   a. If so, how old were the animals?

   b. What were the results?

   c. What are the perceived risks to children based on the results observed in the juvenile animals?

Additional Questions You Might Want to Ask If Your Child Has a Rare Disease

In addition to the aforementioned questions, additional questions should be asked if your child has a rare or serious disease or unmet medical need. Specific issues to take into account when participating in clinical trials if a rare disease is involved are described in Chapter 12.

1. Will this clinical trial involve a biological agent?

   a. If so, what precautions are in place to ensure that side effects are monitored during the clinical trial?

b. If so, what precautions are in place to ensure that possible long-term side effects are monitored after the clinical trial is completed?

2. Were allergic reactions observed in the animal studies that might indicate the potential for allergic reactions during the clinical trial?

3. How many pediatric research subjects will be enrolled in the clinical trial?

4. How many other studies have already been carried out in this program?

5. How long will it take for this clinical trial to be completed, and when will its report be made available?

6. How many additional studies need to be carried out before this drug can be submitted for marketing authorization?

7. Have there been any life-threatening adverse events that could have been related to the drug under study?

References

Committee for Medicinal Products for Human Use (CHMP). (2006). *Guideline on clinical trials in small populations.* CHMP/EWP/83561/2005. Retrieved December 31, 2009, from http://www.emea.europa.eu/pdfs/human/ewp/8356105en.pdf

European Medicines Agency (EMEA), Committee for Medicinal Products for Human Use (CHMP). (2006). *Concept paper on the impact of lung and heart immaturity when investigating medicinal products intended for neonatal use.* EMEA/CHMP/114218/2006. http://www.ama.europa.eu/pdfs/human/paediatrics/11421806en.pdf

European Medicines Agency (EMEA), Committee for Medicinal Products for Human Use (CHMP), Safety Working Party (SWP). (2006). *Role of pharmacokinetics in the development of medicinal products in the paediatric population.* EMEA/CHMP/EWP/147013/2004. Retrieved December 31, 2009, from http://www.emea.europa.eu/pdfs/human/ewp/14701304en.pdf

European Medicines Agency. (2007). *Guideline on the investigation of medicinal products in the term and preterm neonates.* EMEA/267484/2007. Retrieved December 31, 2009, from http://www.emea.europa.eu/pdfs/human/paediatrics/26748407en.pdf

European Medicines Agency (EMEA), Committee for Medicinal Products for Human Use (CHMP), Safety Working Party (SWP). (2008). *Guideline on the need for non-clinical testing in juvenile animals on human pharmaceuticals for paediatric indications.* EMEA/CHMP/SWP/1169215/2005. Retrieved December 31, 2009, from http://www.emea.europa.eu/pdfs/human/swp/16921505en08.pdf

European Parliament and the Council. (2006a). Regulation EC No. 1901 /2006 on Medicinal Products for Pediatric Use. *Official Journal of the European Union, L378*, 1–19.

European Parliament and the Council. (2006b) Regulation (EC) No. 1902/2006 on Medicinal Products for Pediatric Use. *Official Journal of the European Union, l378*, 20–21.

European Parliament and the Council (2007). *Submission of pediatric studies according to Articles 45 & 46 of the Regulation of the European Parliament and of the Council (EC) No. 1901/2006, As amended (Pediatric Regulation).*

International Conference of Harmonization. (2000). *Clinical investigation of medicinal products in the pediatric population.* E11, Step 4.

http://www.ich.org/LOB/media/MEDIA487.pdf.

U. S. Department of Health and Human Services, Food and Drug Administration, Center for Drug Evaluation and Research (CDER), Center for Biologics Evaluation and Research (CBER). (1998). *Guidance for industry—General considerations for pediatric pharmacokinetic studies for drugs and biologics. Draft guidance.* Rockville, MD: Author.

U. S. Department of Health and Human Services, Food and Drug Administration, Center for Drug Evaluation and Research (CDER), Center for Biologics Evaluation and Research (CBER). (1999). *Guidance for industry—Qualifying for pediatric exclusivity under section 505A of the Federal Food, Drug and Cosmetic Act.* Rockville, MD: Author.

U. S. Department of Health and Human Services, Food and Drug Administration, Center for Drug Evaluation and Research (CDER), Center for Biologics

Evaluation and Research (CBER). (2000). *Guidance for industry, E11 clinical investigation of medicinal products in the pediatric population.* Rockville, MD: Author.

U. S. Department of Health and Human Services, Food and Drug Administration. (2001). 21 CFR Parts 50 & 56, Docket No. 00N-0074. *Additional safeguards for children in clinical investigations of FDA regulated products.* Federal Register, April 24, 2001, 66(79), Rules and Regulations, pp. 20589–20600.

U. S. Department of Health and Human Services, Food and Drug Administration, Center for Drug Evaluation and Research (CDER), Center for Biologics Evaluation and Research (CBER). (2005). *Guidance for industry—How to comply with the Pediatric Research Equity Act, Draft Guidance.* Rockville, MD: Author.

U. S. Department of Health and Human Services, Food and Drug Administration, Center for Drug Evaluation and Research (CDER). (2006). *Guidance for industry—Nonclinical safety evaluation of pediatric drug products.* Rockville, MD: Author.

Clinical Trials Involving Rare or Orphan Diseases

12

An orphan disease is a disease that has a relatively small prevalence. These diseases are known as orphan diseases because of the lack of incentive to develop drugs for these therapeutic areas; the patient numbers are too small to provide the payback that encourages sponsors to invest in drug development. The exact number of patients with a disease that leads to it being classified as an orphan disease can vary from country to country. In the United States, that number is less than 200,000 patients. In the European Union, orphan medicines are defined as those intended for the diagnosis, prevention, or treatment of life-threatening or chronically debilitating conditions that affect no more than 5 in 10,000 people in the European Union, or are medicines that, for economic reasons, would be unlikely to be developed without incentives.

Orphan diseases are often life-threatening or chronically debilitating conditions. Many affect children. Because orphan diseases occur in relatively small numbers of patients, it is often the case that very little is known about the disease. Consequently, companies may have to spend a great deal of money learning about the disease before a drug can be discovered and developed. Clearly, there is a need to encourage the development of drugs for these diseases.

To encourage the development of drugs for orphan diseases, governments began to offer incentives, such as data exclusivity, grants, and free advice in the 1980s. Data exclusivity and other incentives give companies the opportunity to market the drugs without competition for specific periods of time, so that they may recuperate their costs more quickly than if these incentives were not available. These incentives also include tax breaks. Some diseases that have benefited from these initiatives include Type 1 Gaucher disease, Fabry disease, mucopolysaccharidosis I, and Pompe disease.

The Regulatory Environment

The major regulatory authorities have introduced regulations and guidelines to assist companies that are developing drugs for orphan diseases (Committee for Orphan Medicinal Products, 2007; European Medicines Agency, 2007; Orphan Drug Regulations, 1992). The number of drugs marketed for orphan diseases has increased significantly after the major regulatory authorities implemented initiatives to encourage development of orphan drugs. For instance, the regulatory environment in Europe now provides opportunities for companies to seek regulatory approval through a special mechanism called "exceptional circumstances" if it would be unethical to repeat an already existent study (Committee for Medicinal Products for Human Use, 2005). Because of the difficulty of conducting studies in orphan indications, approval under "exceptional circumstances" may be applicable for orphan diseases.

The Challenges of Conducting Clinical Trials in Orphan Diseases

There are unique challenges for companies that are carrying out clinical trials in orphan diseases. One of these challenges is that the numbers of patients with the disease can be very small. When those who meet the inclusion and exclusion criteria are considered, the numbers can be further reduced. For diseases with a very small prevalence, the clinical trials may need to be carried out in many countries to ensure sufficient numbers of research subjects can be enrolled in the study to meet the study's objectives. Conducting studies in different countries increases the costs of these studies.

Clinical trials involving relatively small numbers of subjects sometimes require different study designs and approaches not usually used for other disease areas. These studies can take longer to conduct because there may be long gaps of time of months and even years between the enrollment of each patient, depending on the rarity of the disease. Bear in mind that because orphan disease studies are smaller and can take longer to complete, you may not hear about the outcome of the clinical trial for a long time after you participated in a clinical trial involving the study of an orphan disease.

What Should I Do If I Have a Child Who Has a Rare Disease?

Children with rare diseases face the usual challenges faced by children generally (see Chapter 11). For instance, children are unable to give informed consent on their own behalf; their parents or guardians must do that for them. Chapter 11 provides some guidance regarding pediatric clinical trials in general. If your child is adequately managed by the therapies that are being prescribed at this time, it may not be appropriate to interrupt this treatment to place your child in a clinical trial. There may be study designs in which your child could continue on his or her current treatment but also receive the drug under study. If your child's condition is not adequately controlled with currently available drugs, it might be appropriate to try to find clinical trials that are being conducted for the disease your child is suffering from. In the United States, the government Web site http://www.clinicaltrials.gov is a good source of information on ongoing clinical trials. Examples of the types of questions to ask if your child has a rare disease are provided in Chapter 11.

What Should I Do If I Am a Patient with a Rare Disease?

If you have a rare disease and feel you are not being adequately treated, you can conduct a search on the Internet for clinical trials for your disease. If you locate a clinical trial, you should discuss the study with your general practitioner. Your general practitioner will be familiar with your medical history and may be aware of reasons why a particular study may or may not be suitable for you. If your general practitioner believes you are a good candidate for the clinical trial, he or she may be able to refer you to the principal investigator (PI) by means of a telephone call and/or letter. In some countries, referrals to PIs will need to be made by general practitioners. Victor found it helpful to involve his general practitioner in his evaluation of a clinical trial.

Victor's Story

Victor is a 40-year-old man who is suffering from a very rare condition, which is an orphan disease. There is currently no cure for his disease, although his condition is controlled by treating his symptoms. After conducting an Internet search for a clinical trial, he has found a clinical trial targeted to his disease, but it is being carried out in another part of the country. He is very excited about what he has read about the clinical trial results. The drug is in Phase 3, and it is being evaluated in patients in several different countries. So far 30 research subjects have been dosed with the drug in Phase 3. Victor would need to drive or fly to the part of the country where research subjects are being enrolled into the clinical trial, several times per month, during the clinical trial. He decides to discuss the clinical trial with his general practitioner. The general practitioner carries out his own research into the clinical trial, carefully evaluating the published results. He confirms that 30 research subjects have been enrolled into the clinical trial so far, that the study has been ongoing for 4 years, and that recruitment is taking place in 10 countries.

The general practitioner offers to write a letter of referral to the PI on Victor's behalf. The PI agrees to evaluate Victor for enrollment into the clinical trial. Victor travels to the investigative site on two occasions and is eventually enrolled into the clinical trial. The sponsor of the clinical trial has agreed to pay Victor's expenses so that he can take part in the clinical trial.

Points to Consider

1. It was appropriate for Victor to discuss the clinical trial results with his general practitioner, who could objectively examine the results available in the scientific literature for the drug.

2. Although only 30 research subjects have so far been enrolled in the Phase 3 program, the total number required to show efficacy may not be large because the disease is very rare.

3. The general practitioner was able to initiate a dialogue with the PI to ensure that Victor was a suitable candidate for the clinical trial, saving Victor a wasted journey to the investigative site.

4. Victor will be able to take part in the clinical trial with the reassurance that he has made a good decision with the help of his general practitioner.

Research subjects with genetic illnesses, which may also be rare, may need to consider the implications (for their relatives who may also have the disease or may be carriers of the disease) of their enrollment in clinical trials that involve genetic testing. Denise spent quite a lot of time thinking about this before enrolling in a clinical trial involving the study of her rare inherited disease.

Denise's Story

Denise is a young woman with a rare genetic disease. She wants to contribute to the body of knowledge about her illness for her own sake and to benefit future generations of her family who may also inherit this disease. She contacted the National Institutes of Health and found a clinical trial in which she could participate. She attended the investigative site for an assessment visit. It appeared that she would meet all the inclusion and exclusion criteria based on her health status. She was informed that the study was a Phase 2 study and was producing some good results based on the doses observed to be safe during the Phase 1 studies.

Points to Consider

1. If Denise has to travel a long distance to the investigative site, she should make enquiries about who will pay the travel expenses.
2. Denise may be given genetic testing during the clinical trial. The implications of the knowledge gained regarding the rest of her family who are genetically related to her, and how to deal with the information gained, should be considered carefully at the outset as she determines whether to take part in the clinical trial.

Some Questions You Might Want to Ask If You or Your Child Has a Rare Disease

1. Will this clinical trial be spread across several different countries? If yes, how long will it take for the clinical trial to be completed and the results to be published?
2. When is it anticipated that the drug may be registered?
3. When is it anticipated that the drug may be commercialized?
4. How many additional studies need to be carried out before this drug may be submitted for marketing authorization?
5. Will this clinical trial involve a biological agent?
   a. If so, what precautions are in place to ensure that side effects are monitored during the clinical trial?
   b. If so, what precautions are in place to ensure that possible long-term side effects are monitored after the clinical trial is completed?
6. Were allergic reactions observed in the animal studies that might indicate the potential for allergic reactions during the clinical trial?
7. How many research subjects will be enrolled in the clinical trial?
8. How many other studies have already been carried out in this program?
9. Have there been any life-threatening adverse events that were considered related to the drug?

References

Committee for Medicinal Products for Human Use (CHMP). (2005). *Guideline on procedures for the granting of a marketing authorisation under exceptional circumstances, pursuant to Article 14 (8) of Regulation (EC) No. 726/2004.* EMEA/357981/2005. Retrieved December 31, 2009, from http://www.emea.europa.eu/pdfs/human/euleg/35798105en.pdf

Committee for Orphan Medicinal Products (COMP). (2002). *Points to consider on the calculation and reporting of the prevalence of a condition for orphan designation.* COMP/436/01. Retrieved December 31, 2009, from http://www.emea.europa.eu/pdfs/human/comp/043601.pdf

European Medicines Agency. (2007). *Orphan drugs and rare diseases at a glance.* EMEA/290072/2007. Retrieved December 31, 2009, from http://www.emea.europa.eu/pdfs/human/comp/29007207en.pdf

Orphan Drug Regulation, 21 C. F. R. Part 316: Final Rule [Docket No. 85N-0483], RIN 0905-AB55. (1992).

Clinical Trials Involving Disabled and Vulnerable Groups

An individual should not be prevented from participating in a clinical trial because he or she is physically disabled. However, a sponsor of a clinical trial and those overseeing the clinical trial will need to take special care to ensure that the rights of the individual are carefully considered and protected, depending on the nature of the disability. It is difficult to justify enrolling mentally disabled patients in clinical trials that are complex, and for which they will not be able to give their informed consent, unless the benefits clearly outweigh the risks. Even in situations where a guardian will give informed consent for the research subject in these cases, the ethics of such participation will need to be carefully evaluated by all involved.

In accordance with the Declaration of Helsinki, no one should be forced to enter a clinical trial. Clinical protocols that are to be conducted in a vulnerable population must go through a rigorous ethical review by the ethics committee (EC). If you are related to someone whom you consider vulnerable and whom you believe is being coerced into a clinical trial or who cannot adequately give informed consent, this should be reported to the EC (see Chapter 3). In these cases, a patient advocate may be assigned. In situations where the patient's interests cannot be represented adequately, the clinical trial situation is not appropriate.

Clinical Trials Involving the Disabled

There are many different types of disabilities. A person may be born disabled, or the person may develop a disability as a result of an illness. As an illness progresses in its severity, the level of disability may also worsen. Some clinical trials may be carried out specifically in the disabled. In these situations, arrangements such as additional support may be needed to ensure that the disability in question is not an impediment to participation in the clinical trial. At other times, because the protocol and clinical trial logistics were planned with able-bodied research subjects in mind, additional arrangements may need to be made to ensure that the disabled research subject is able to participate if he or she otherwise meets the inclusion and exclusion criteria. Some of these principles are illustrated by Jonathan's story.

Jonathan's Story

Jonathan is a 25-year-old young man who suffered a brain trauma during birth. He is cared for by his loving parents. Physicians have told his parents that he does not know them, but they believe differently. Two years ago he developed a wound on his leg that has not healed. The physician informed Jonathan's parents about a clinical trial involving a new dressing that would involve daily administration in the home environment and weekly visits to the investigative site for evaluation. His parents are pleased that there is a new dressing under evaluation that may help their son's condition.

Points to Consider

1. Because Jonathan is mentally disabled, he cannot give his informed consent. His parents are very loving and are therefore likely to make a decision that is in his best interest. They can give informed consent on his behalf because they are his guardians.

2. Jonathan's parents can ask for a patient advocate to advise them in evaluating the information available about the clinical trial. This will help to ensure that this trial is the best clinical trial for their son and that other commercially available alternatives would not be better for his wound care.

3. It would be appropriate to determine if Jonathan will experience any discomfort as a result of the wound dressing procedure.

4. His parents should also seek to determine how many other research subjects have entered the clinical trial and what the results have been so far. The principal investigator (PI) may not be able to divulge the clinical trial results gathered to that point if the study is conducted in a double-blind fashion.

Clinical Trials Involving the Hearing Impaired and Deaf

Sign language experts and interpreters can be requested by the clinical trial staff. These can be requested for a particular research subject on an as-needed basis. Arrangements should be made in advance to ensure that the sign language experts are available for each visit when the research subject attends for study follow-ups. The PI should arrange for the sign language expert to be trained on the study materials. This will ensure that the research subject is given the appropriate information and that there are no misinterpretations or misunderstandings.

Clinical Trials Involving the Blind

If a research subject is blind, it is clear that extra arrangements will need to be made to transport that individual to the investigative site for visits. Additional support will need to be arranged to ensure that the research subject receives materials about the clinical trial in Braille. A patient advocate and a staff of nurses and study coordinators will need to work with the research subject to ensure that support is available on a daily basis to assure compliance with the study procedures. Although these additional provisions will add to the cost of conducting the study, the sponsor should not turn a research subject away because he or she is blind if the subject otherwise meets the inclusion/exclusion criteria. Sufficient time will need to be allowed for the support and materials to be put into place. Randomization to the investigational drug group or the placebo group must be done in such a way that bias is not introduced into the clinical trial; all materials will need to be prepared in Braille regardless of the group to which the patient is randomized. Let us see how Phillip, a blind man with diabetes, will handle the clinical trial situation.

Phillip's Story

Phillip has been blind since birth. He is 52 years old and somewhat overweight. Two years ago he was diagnosed with type 2 diabetes. His diabetes has been difficult to control. His physician, a diabetes specialist, has changed his medication on three occasions. Phillip either experiences unacceptable side effects or becomes hypoglycemic while taking them. His specialist has heard about a clinical trial to study a new antidiabetic medication that has been producing good results. The drug is now in late-stage Phase 3 studies. If Phillip can be accepted in the clinical trial, this drug might eventually provide a good alternative for the treatment of his diabetes. His specialist made a referral to the PI and arranged for Phillip to be seen at the investigative site for an evaluation to see if he would meet the inclusion/exclusion criteria.

The PI evaluated Phillip for entry in the clinical trial. He met all the inclusion and exclusion criteria. The PI arranged for the informed consent document to be printed in Braille. He also arranged for a patient advocate to be assigned to him.

The patient advocate will be able to ensure that Phillip understands the clinical trial enough to give his informed consent. The patient advocate will also be able to ensure that Phillip is comfortable with the information presented in Braille.

Points to Consider

1. The fact that Phillip is blind does not mean that he cannot be included in a clinical trial.
2. It was appropriate that the specialist with knowledge of his medical condition made the referral to the PI.
3. The patient advocate will be able to ensure that Phillip is adequately supported as he participates in the clinical trial.

Clinical Trials Involving the Mentally Ill

Patients who have psychiatric illnesses or who are otherwise mentally ill are prescribed and administered many medicines. Some of these medicines are for the psychiatric illness, and others are for physiological illnesses. Psychiatric medicines have to be tested in those who are mentally ill. Because of the need for a research subject to be able to give informed consent, the patients with mild to moderate psychiatric disease may tend to be studied in the clinical trial setting. If patients are unable to give their informed consent, serious consideration must be given to the appropriateness of entering them in a clinical trial, especially if other licensed medicines are available to treat them. After marketing, patients with very severe illness may experience problems with these medications because they were not represented in the clinical trials. This is one of the practical difficulties of dealing with mental illness in a clinical trial setting.

In the United States, the National Institute of Mental Health (NIMH) is a part of the National Institutes of Health. This organization conducts clinical trials in patients with mental illness. These studies are carried out in Bethesda, Maryland, near Washington, DC. Expenses for transportation to the investigative site are usually reimbursed by the National Institutes of Mental Health. Some mental illnesses as defined by the NIMH are as shown in Table 13.1.

Table 13.1 Some Mental Illnesses That Can be Studied in Clinical Trials

Mental Illnesses
Anxiety disorders
Attention-deficit/hyperactivity disorder (ADHD, ADD)
Autism spectrum disorders (pervasive developmental disorders)
Bipolar disorders (manic depressive illnesses)
Borderline personality disorder
Depression
Eating disorders
Generalized anxiety disorder
Obsessive-compulsive disorder (OCD)
Panic disorder
Schizophrenia
Social phobia (social anxiety disorder)
Conditions Related to Mental Disorders
Perimenopausal-related mood disorders
Postpartum depression
Posttraumatic stress disorder
Premenstrual syndrome

Other Types of Vulnerable Research Subjects

There are many types of vulnerable patients that I have not specifically described in this chapter. The guiding principle must be that the dignity, safety, and respect for the individual are paramount over the need of a sponsor to conduct a clinical trial in a particular patient group.

Where a patient advocate is unable to assist a research subject in understanding the clinical trial, a PI and a sponsor should err on the side of caution and not include the research subject in the clinical trial. However, difficult situations must be managed and overcome so that research subjects with disabilities can be enrolled in clinical trials if they will derive benefit from this participation and if they meet the inclusion/exclusion criteria. Contingency plans should exist so that the necessary adjustments can be made to enable disabled research subjects to enter and participate in clinical trials. The ethical standards that apply to these patients are the same as for research subjects that do not have disabilities. Additional safeguards may need to be put in place to ensure that the rights of the research subject are safeguarded under these conditions, depending on the country in which the clinical trial is taking place.

Questions to Ask the Principal Investigator and Study Staff If You Are Disabled

1. Will I experience any particular difficulties in taking part in the clinical trial with my particular disability?
2. Will I need any special support services to ensure that I can take part in this specific clinical trial?

Questions to Ask the Principal Investigator and Study Staff If You Represent Someone Who Is Disabled

1. Do you foresee any particular difficulties during the clinical trial for someone with these disabilities?
2. What sort of support will be provided to assist someone with these disabilities?
3. What can I do to provide adequate support during the clinical trial?

Some Helpful Resources

14

There is a wealth of information available to you as a potential participant in a clinical trial. Some of this information is disease specific, and other information is related to the clinical trial process. Books, journals, magazines, the Internet, and patient advocacy groups are good sources of information about clinical trials. It is not feasible for all available resources to be listed in this chapter, but a limited number are included. You can contact the librarian at your local library for assistance in finding information regarding clinical trials for your disease area, as well as if you need information about your specific disease.

If you are already participating in a clinical trial, there will be a lot of information available to you about the specific clinical trial from the investigative site. The sponsor of the clinical trial is also a good source of information and likely has a Web site. The sponsor will make information available to you via the principal investigator (PI), but cannot provide you with any information that may introduce bias into the study or potentially affect the study outcome. Making direct contact with the sponsor's medical information department may enable you to locate suitable clinical trials. However, bear in mind that the sponsor cannot address questions about your medical condition. All requests for disease-specific information should go through your general practitioner if you are not enrolled in a clinical trial, or the PI if you are.

The Internet is an important source of information on clinical trials. Well-known hospital and clinic institutions post information about clinical trials that are planned and ongoing on their Web sites. You can check these regularly to find information.

The Food and Drug Administration requires that sponsors of clinical trials post information about their studies on the government Web site: http://www.clinicaltrials.gov. You should check this Web site as a starting point for information about ongoing clinical trials in your disease area if you live in the United States. This Web site also provides information on the clinical trial process that you might find helpful.

Local magazines and newspapers can be good sources of information about clinical trials. Local radio stations are also used by clinical research organizations (CROs) to advertise for upcoming and ongoing studies that are looking for participants. Notice boards in grocery stores may list local clinical trials. The sponsors of clinical trials are very innovative about locating potential research subjects for their clinical trials; you may hear or see requests for patients to contact sponsors or clinical research organizations in many places.

Where to Find Information on Clinical Trials

The Internet search engines such as Google and Yahoo can be used to find the information that you are looking for regarding clinical trials.

You will need to input keywords to narrow the search. Some suggested keywords are as follows:

"Clinical trials"
"Clinical trials for INSERT DISEASE NAME"
"Patient advocacy"
"Patient advocacy INSERT DISEASE NAME"
Web sites dedicated to disease areas—for example, "hypertension," "type 1 diabetes," "type 2 diabetes"
Web sites for hospital and investigative sites—for example, "Mayo Clinic," "UCLA," "MD Anderson"
Company or sponsor Web sites
Physician office Web sites

You can input any search term or combination of search terms to find the information you are looking for.

Some Web Sites for General Information or to Find Clinical Trials

http://www.clinicaltrials.gov—this Web site is the official US government list of clinical trials
http://www.searchclinicaltrials.org—a good resource for finding clinical trials
http://www.centerwatch.com—clinical trial resources, including listings
http://www.cancer.gov—resources for cancer clinical trials
http://www.nlm.nih.gov/medlineplus/clinicaltrials.html—this Web site provides tutorials and information on clinical trials
http://www.nimh.nih.gov/health/trials/index.shtml—mental health clinical trials
http://www.cancer.org—resources regarding cancer clinical trials

http://www.aidsinfo.nih.gov/ClinicalTrials/Default.aspx—clinical trial resources for those with HIV/AIDS

http://www.fda.gov/oashi/clinicaltrials/default.htm—FDA resources regarding the clinical trial process

http://www.fda.gov/oc/gcp/default.htm—information on good clinical practice

https://www.actgnetwork.org—clinical trials in acquired immune deficiency syndrome (AIDS) http://www.fda.gov/oashi/clinicaltrials/default.htm—Regulatory updates on clinical trials in HIV/AIDS.

http://www.pubmed.com—a Web site for finding scientific publications

http://www.fda.gov/oc/ohrt/irbs/default.htm—information on institutional review boards

http://www.fda.gov/oc/ohrt/irbs/faqs.htm—information on institutional review boards

http://www.hhs.gov/ohrp/—Office for Human Research Protections

http://www.fda.gov/cdrh—information regarding devices

http://www.fda.gov/cber/—regulatory information regarding biological products

http://www.nih.gov/—National Institutes of Health information regarding clinical trials

http://www4.od.nih.gov/oba/—National Institutes of Health information regarding gene therapy clinical research

Resources for the United Kingdom

http://www.cancerhelp.org.uk/trials/trials/—finding clinical trials in the United Kingdom

For research subjects in other European countries, you can ask your local librarian for information on resources or conduct a search on the Internet using Google or another search engine.

Experimental and Gene Therapy Clinical Trials

http://www.fda.gov/cber/gene.htm—information regarding gene transfer experiments

http://www4.od.nih.gov/oba—information regarding gene transfer clinical research

Information Regarding Xenotransplantation

http://www.fda.gov/biologics/xenotransplantation/default.htm

Books

The following are suggested books for further reading. This list is far from exhaustive. You can search for additional reading resources at http://www.google.com using appropriate search terms or by searching under http://www.amazon.com.

Inlander, C. B., & Weiner, E. (1997). *Take this book to the hospital with you*. Allentown, PA: People's Medical Society.

Keene, N. (1998). *Working with your doctor: Getting the healthcare you deserve*. Cambridge, MA: O'Reilly & Associates.

Oster, N., Thomas, L., & Joseff, D. (2000). *Making informed medical decisions: Where to look and how to use what you find*. Sebastopol, CA: O'Reilly & Associates.

Soden, K. J., & Dumas, C. (2003). *Special treatment: How to get the same high-quality health care your doctor gets*. New York: Berkley Books.

Zakarian, B. (1996). *The activist cancer patient: How to take charge of your treatment*. New York: John Wiley & Sons.

Addresses and Web Sites for Patient Support and Advocacy Groups

Table 14.1 lists addresses and Web sites for patient support and advocacy groups in the United States. These groups will usually be aware of the clinical trials that are ongoing for specific disease areas. This list is not exhaustive. Additional advocacy groups can be found by searching on http://www.google.com using the disease terms with the search term "advocacy" or "patient support." Advocacy groups based in the US may be aware of equivalent advocacy groups in other countries. Groups for your specific country can be found on the Internet or at your local library by using your country as a search term with the terms "disease" and "support" or "advocacy group": for example, "diabetes" and "advocacy group" and "country name." Your librarian will be able to find support and/or advocacy groups that are active for the disease area which is relevant for you.

Table 14.1 Patient Support and Advocacy Groups

Cancer Groups	
Action to Cure Kidney Cancer 150 West 75th St. Suite 246 New York, NY 10023	http://www.ackc.org
American Cancer Society 1599 Clifton Rd, NE Atlanta, GA 30329	http://www.cancer.org
Alliance for Prostate Cancer Prevention 15248 South Tamiami Trail Suite 1000 Fort Myers, FL 33908	http://www.APCaP.org
Brain Tumor Society 124 Watertown Street, Suite 3H Watertown, MA 02472	http://www.tbts.org
West Coast Office 22 Battery Street, Suite 612 San Francisco, CA 94111-5520	
Cancer Care, Inc. 275 Seventh Ave. Floor 22 New York, NY 10001	http://www.cancercare.org
Cancer Research and Prevention Foundation 1600 Duke Street Suite 500 Alexandria, VA 22314	http://www.preventcancer.org

The Childhood Brain Tumor Foundation 20312 Watkins Meadow Drive Germantown, MD 20876	http://www.childhoodbraintumor.org
Children's Cause for Cancer Advocacy, Inc. 1010 Wayne Avenue, Suite 770 Silver Spring, MD 20910	http://www.childrenscause.org
Colon Cancer Alliance 1200 G Street, NW Suite 800 Washington, DC 20005	http://www.ccalliance.org
Colorectal Cancer Association of Canada 5 Place Ville Marie, Suite 1230 Montréal, Quebec Canada H3B 2G2	http://www.ccac-accc.ca
Colorectal Cancer Association of Canada 60 St. Clair Avenue East Suite 204 Toronto, Ontario Canada M4T 1N5	http://www.ccac-accc.ca
Cancer Network	http://www.cancernetwork.com Information about different cancers is available at the above Web site
Georgia Center for Oncology Research & Education (GA-CORE) 50 Hurt Plaza, Suite 704 Atlanta, GA 30303	http://www.gacore.org
GIST (Gastrointestinal Stromal Tumor) Support International 12 Bomaca Drive Doylestown, PA 18901	http://www.gistsupport.org
International Cancer Advocacy Network 27 West Morten Avenue Phoenix, AZ 85021-7246	http://www.askican.org
International Myeloma Foundation 12650 Riverside Drive, Suite 206 North Hollywood, CA 91607-3421	http://www.myeloma.org
Joe's House 50 Lexington Avenue Suite 10H New York, NY 10010	http://www.joeshouse.org

*Joe's House is a nonprofit organization providing a
nationwide online service that helps cancer patients and
their families find lodging near treatment centers.*

(*continued*)

Table 14.1 Patient Support and Advocacy Groups (*continued*)

Cancer Groups	
Kidney Cancer Association	http://www.kidneycancerassociation.org

Canada
Postal letters only, please
207-1425 Marine Drive
West Vancouver, BC
Canada V7T 1B9

European Union
Postal letters only, please
2nd floor
145-157 St. John Street
London EC1V 4PY

Washington, DC
Postal letters only, please
PO Box 96503
Washington, DC 20090

Lance Armstrong Foundation	http://www.laf.org
P O Box 161150	
Austin, TX 78716-1150	
Lung Cancer Alliance	http://www.lungcanceralliance.org
888 16th St, NW	
Suite 150	
Washington, DC 20006	
Lung Cancer Circle of Hope	http://www.lungcancercircleofhope.org
Lung Cancer Circle of Hope	
7 Carnation Drive, Suite A	
Lakewood, NJ 08701	
Lymphoma Research Foundation	http://www.lymphoma.org

New York Office
115 Broadway, 13th Floor
New York, NY 10006

Los Angeles Office
8800 Venice Blvd, Suite 207
Los Angeles, CA 90034

The Lustgarten Foundation for	http://www.lustgartenfoundation.org
Pancreatic Cancer Research	
1111 Stewart Avenue	
Bethpage, New York 11714	

Melanoma Research Foundation
The Melanoma Research Foundation
170 Township Line Road, Bldg B
Hillsborough, NJ 08844

http://www.melanoma.org

Multiple Myeloma Research Foundation
383 Main Avenue
5th floor
Norwalk, CT 06851

http://www.multiplemyeloma.org

National Brain Tumor Foundation

http://www.braintumor.org

East Coast Office

124 Watertown Street, Suite 2D
Watertown, MA 02472

West Coast Office

22 Battery Street, Suite 612
San Francisco, CA 94111-5520

National Coalition for Cancer Survivorship
1010 Wayne Avenue
Suite 770
Silver Spring, MD 20910

http://www.canceradvocacy.org

National Lymphedema Network
Latham Square
1611 Telegraph Avenue, Suite 1111
Oakland, CA 94612-2138

http://www.lymphnet.org

National Ovarian Cancer Coalition, Inc.
2501 Oak Lawn Avenue
Suite 435
Dallas, TX 75219

http://www.ovarian.org

National Patient Advocate Foundation
725 15th St. NW, 10th Floor
Washington, DC 20005

http://www.npaf.org

ZERO—The Project to End Prostate Cancer
10 G Street NE, Suite 601
Washington, DC 20002

http://www.zerocancer.org

Ovarian Cancer National Alliance
910 17th Street, NW, Suite 1190
Washington, DC 20006

http://www.ovariancancer.org

Pancreatic Cancer Action Network
2141 Rosecrans Ave., Suite 7000
El Segundo, CA 90245

http://www.pancan.org

(*continued*)

Table 14.1 Patient Support and Advocacy Groups (*continued*)

Cancer Groups

Pennsylvania Breast Cancer Coalition Statewide Headquarters Trout Run Business Center 344 North Reading Road Ephrata, PA 17522	http://www.pabreastcancer.org
Research Advocacy Network 6505 W Park Blvd, Suite 305, PMB 220 Plano, TX 75093	http://www.researchadvocacy.org
Sarcoma Alliance 775 East Blithedale, #334 Mill Valley, CA 94941	http://www.sarcomaalliance.org
Sarcoma Foundation of America 9884 Main Street P.O. Box 458 Damascus, MD 20872	http://www.curesarcoma.org
Skin Cancer Foundation Madison Avenue, Suite 901 New York, NY 10016	http://www.skincancer.org
Support for People with Oral and Head and Neck Cancer PO Box 53 Locust Valley, NY 11560-0053	http://www.spohnc.org
Susan G. Komen Breast Cancer Foundation Headquarters 5005 LBJ Freeway, Suite 250 Dallas, TX 75244	http://ww5.komen.org
The Life Raft Group The Life Raft Group (A GIST support group) 40 Galesi Drive Wayne, NJ 07470	http://www.liferaftgroup.org
Us Too! Prostate Cancer Education and Support 5003 Fairview Avenue Downers Grove, IL 60515	http://www.ustoo.com
Vital Options International Inc. 4419 Coldwater Canyon Ave., Suite I Studio City, CA 91604-1479	http://www.vitaloptions.org
Wellness Community 919 18th Street NW, Suite 54 Washington, DC 20006	http://www.thewellnesscommunity.org

Yul Brynner Head and Neck Cancer Foundation, Inc. 135 Rutledge Ave. MSC 550 Charleston, SC 29425-5500	http://www.headandneck.org
American Brain Tumor Association 2720 River Road Des Plaines, IL 60018	http://www.abta.org

Alzheimer Disease Groups

Alzheimer's Association **National office** 225 N. Michigan Ave., Fl. 17 Chicago, IL 60601-7633	http://www.alz.org

Asthma Groups

American Academy of Allergy, Asthma & Immunology 555 East Wells Street Suite 1100 Milwaukee, WI 53202-3823	http://www.aaaai.org

Bone

The Paget Foundation 120 Wall Street, Suite 1602 New York, NY 10005-4001	http://www.paget.org

Diabetes Groups

National Diabetes Information Clearinghouse 1 Information Way Bethesda, MD 20892–3560	http://diabetes.niddk.nih.gov
American Diabetes Association ATTN: National Call Center 1701 North Beauregard Street Alexandria, VA 22311	http://www.diabetes.org

HIV/AIDS Groups

American Foundation for AIDS Research 733 3rd Ave 12th Floor New York, NY 10017	http://www.amfar.org

(*continued*)

Table 14.1 Patient Support and Advocacy Groups (*continued*)

Cancer Groups

Pediatric AIDS Foundation   http://www.pedaids.org

Washington, DC
1140 Connecticut Avenue NW
Suite 200
Washington, DC 20036

Los Angeles, CA
11150 Santa Monica Blvd.
Suite 1050
Los Angeles, CA 90025

Côte D'Ivoire
2 Plateau Neighborhood
Blocks A & C, 3rd Floor
Abidjan, Côte D'Ivoire

Kenya
ABC Place, 4th Floor Waiyaki Way
PO Box 13612-00800
Nairobi, Kenya

Dermatology Groups

American Skin Association   http://www.americanskin.org
346 Park Avenue South
New York, NY 10010

Dermatology Foundation   http://www.dermatologyfoundation.org
1560 Sherman Ave.
Evanston, IL 60201-4802

National Eczema Society   http://www.eczema.org
163 Eversholt St
London NW1 1BU,
United Kingdom

Gastrointestinal Groups

Crohn's and Colitis Foundation of America   http://www.ccfa.org
386 Park Avenue South
17th Floor
New York, NY 10016

Hematology Groups

Sickle Cell Disease Association of America, Inc.   http://www.sicklecelldisease.org
231 East Baltimore Street
Suite 800
Baltimore, MD 21202

Mental Health Groups

Mental Health America
2000 N. Beauregard Street,
6th Floor Alexandria, VA 22311

http://www.mentalhealthamerica.net

National Institute of Mental Health (NIMH)
Science Writing, Press, and
Dissemination Branch
6001 Executive Blvd,
Room 8184, MSC 9663
Bethesda, MD 20892-9663

http://www.nimh.nih.gov

Miscellaneous Groups

Patient Advocate Foundation
700 Thimble Shoals Blvd, Suite 200, Newport
News, VA 23606

http://www.patientadvocate.org

Celiac Disease Foundation
13251 Ventura Blvd, Number 3
Studio City, CA 91604-1838

http://www.celiac.org

Sjögren's Syndrome Foundation
6707 Democracy Blvd
Suite 325
Bethesda, MD 20817

http://www.sjogrens.org

Ophthalmology Groups

American Macular Degeneration Foundation
P.O. Box 515
Northampton, MA 01061-0515

http://www.macular.org

The Foundation Fighting Blindness
11435 Cronhill Drive
Owings Mills, MD 21117-2220

http://www.blindness.org

Rare Diseases Groups

National Organization for Rare Disorders (NORD)
P.O. Box 8923
New Fairfield, CT 06812-8923

http://www.rarediseases.org/

Office of Rare Diseases Research
National Institutes of Health
6100 Executive Blvd
Room 3B01, MSC 7518
Bethesda, Maryland 20892-7518

http://rarediseases.info.nih.gov

(*continued*)

Table 14.1 Patient Support and Advocacy Groups (*continued*)

Cancer Groups

Rheumatology Groups

Arthritis Foundation P.O. Box 1900 Atlanta, GA 30326	http://www.arthritis.org
National Osteoporosis Foundation 1232 22nd Street NW Washington, DC 20037-1202	http://www.nof.org

---

Systemic Lupus Erythematosus (Lupus) Groups

Lupus Foundation of America, Inc. 4 Research Place, Suite 180 Rockville, MD 20850-3226	http://www.lupus.org

---

Final Thoughts

15

By the time that you have come to the end of this book, I think you will agree that the clinical trial process is a complex one. Perhaps by now you also realize that as a research subject you are an integral, crucial part of the clinical trial process. At no time should you feel intimidated by the complexity of the process nor should you remain silent when you have questions. The professionals that conduct clinical trials are there to serve the research subjects. You should not feel ill at ease as you raise questions or bring issues to the attention of those charged with assuring the safety of the process.

I anticipate that you will have some new questions that may come to mind as you have been reading or as you have personally experienced the clinical trial process. That is to be expected. Throughout this book I have suggested some useful resources to assist you in addressing your questions. Even if all your questions are addressed by this book, you may wish to find out more about how new drugs are developed.

An informed research subject makes a good participant in the clinical research process, so I encourage you to do your own research.

Research subjects have many different types of needs that may influence why they decided to enter clinical trials. If you are seriously ill, your mind may be going in many different directions at the same time, and it may not be reasonable to expect you to absorb a lot of the information presented to you by the physicians and nurses. I hope this book will help you to hone in on the major issues that need your attention. For instance, if you are seriously ill, it is critical that you understand the difference between a Phase 1 clinical trial and a Phase 3 clinical trial. If you are a healthy volunteer, your health should be regarded as your prized possession. It is vital that you ensure that seemingly harmless clinical research does not result in your health being compromised.

Having a sick child is a traumatic experience for the child, the parents, and the family involved. Children diagnosed with rare or incurable diseases may have few other options besides an adequately conducted clinical trial. It behooves the parents or guardians that find themselves in this situation to carefully evaluate the potential for benefit against the risk. In these situations, and in situations involving the terminally or seriously ill, it is vital that experimental clinical research is not presented as treatment to the parents.

Patients with disabilities have the same rights to participate in clinical trials as those who are not disabled. Investigative sites should make appropriate arrangements to accommodate those with disabilities. Therefore, the presence of a disability should not discourage you from finding out more about a clinical trial. Research subjects with disabilities, however, will still need to comply with the protocol in terms of the inclusion and exclusion criteria.

Patients with rare or orphan diseases may find it difficult to find clinical trials for their disease or disorder. In these situations, it is necessary to try to broaden the search to other regions of the country in which you live. The principal investigator conducting the trial in these situations may be able to suggest solutions to ensure enrollment in the clinical trial or availability of the drug in a supervised way.

I sincerely hope that this book has assisted you in your quest for a greater understanding of the clinical trial process. The book set out to make the process less bewildering to research subjects than it must otherwise seem. A process in which the research subjects are informed and therefore empowered will help to ensure the continued availability of new drugs so that diseases that cannot be treated today will be effectively treated tomorrow.

Glossary

This glossary is by no means a comprehensive list of all the jargon and terminology that you might encounter during the clinical trial process. The terms included here have been prepared with the intention of making terms and jargon used in this book understandable; therefore, the definitions provided may not be official textbook definitions. If a term is used during meetings with the clinical investigators or their staff, you should ask for the term to be written down and explained to you. You can then look it up on your own to make sure that you understand it. Scientific dictionaries and the Internet are good sources of information as you conduct your research.

Absorption, distribution, metabolism, and excretion (ADME) The process a drug goes through in the body after it has been administered to an animal or human.

Accrual. *See also* **Enrollment** The process of placing research subjects into a clinical trial. The term also applies to the projected number of research subjects planned for inclusion in a clinical trial.

Active pharmaceutical ingredient (API); Active ingredient The component of a medicine that is pharmacologically active or that produces the medicine's pharmacological effect.

Acute toxicology; Acute toxicity Toxicity that occurs within a short period of time after a single dose or after a single administration of a pharmacologically active agent, usually at a very high dose.

Adenine One of the four bases in DNA, abbreviated as A. Adenine always pairs with thymine. *See also* Base pairs.

Adult stem cells Undifferentiated cell types found among differentiated cells in the organ or in the tissue. They are defined by their origin. Their primary role is to maintain and repair the tissue in which they are found. Although called adult stem cells, they are also present in children.

Adverse drug reaction (ADR) An unfavorable response to a drug.

Adverse effect Any undesired event associated with the administration or use of a medicine or drug.

Adverse event (AE) Any unfavorable medical occurrence that occurs after a drug is administered. It is not necessary to prove that the adverse event is caused by the drug in order for it to be classified as an adverse event. It is only necessary to demonstrate that there is a temporal (time) link to the administration of the drug.

Advocacy group Organizations and groups that actively support participants and their families with valuable resources and advice.

Advocate A person that represents a research subject to ensure that the subject's interests are represented and protected. A relative or family friend may act as an advocate for a research subject.

Alzheimer disease A progressive neurologic disease of the brain that leads to the irreversible loss of neurons and dementia. The clinical hallmarks of Alzheimer disease are progressive impairment in memory, judgment, decision making, orientation to physical surroundings, and language.

Anecdotal Information or data presented to support a particular point of view that often lacks systematic methodology for its collection and support from research.

Approval The affirmative decision by an institutional review board/ethics committee that the clinical trial has been reviewed and may proceed. A decision by a regulatory authority that a clinical trial may proceed or that a drug can be placed on the market.

Audit A systematic and independent review of data and documentation carried out by the Food and Drug Administration, regulatory authorities, or the sponsor. The purpose of a clinical audit is to determine the extent to which the clinical protocols were followed. Audits are used during drug development to determine the extent to which quality standards were followed.

Authorization; Approval The process by which an application to market a drug is granted permission to be commercialized after a detailed process of review. This may also be the process by which a clinical trial is given permission to proceed after a process of review of the documentation.

Autoimmune diseases Diseases in which the body's own immune system attacks its own organs.

Base pairs DNA is made up of bases that pair with each other to form the helical structure. The bases are the "letters" that spell out the genetic code. In DNA, the code letters are A, T, G, and C, which stand for the chemicals adenine, thymine, guanine, and cytosine, respectively. In base pairing, adenine always pairs with thymine, and guanine always pairs with cytosine.

Baseline Measurements taken on a research subject before a drug is administered. The results that are produced after the drug is administered can be compared to those that were present at baseline.

Basic research Research conducted to gain knowledge or understanding of a disease under study. This research advances scientific knowledge, which can be used to develop new drugs.

Belmont Report A US document that establishes the principles and guidelines for the protection of human subjects during research.

Benefit. *See also* **Efficacy** Improvement in the clinical condition from baseline.

Bias A situation in which the results of a study can be influenced to produce a result that would not have been otherwise produced. Results produced when bias is present are unreliable.

Biochemistry The study of the chemical processes that occur in living organisms, including the study of cellular components such as proteins, carbohydrates, lipids, nucleic acids, and other molecules.

Biological agent A drug that is biological, rather than chemical, in nature.

Biosafety committee. *See also* **Institutional biosafety committee (IBC)** An advisory group that reviews the documentation for biological, gene therapy, and experimental therapies in the United States to assure that they are safe enough to be handled by the health care professionals at the investigative site, and that they are safe enough to be administered to research subjects.

Biotechnology A technology that is based on biological research and findings.

Blinded studies. *See also* **Double blind; Single blind** Research in which subjects and/or the investigator are unaware of the treatment that is being administered.

Board certification The process by which a qualified physician undertakes a series of specialized training after which this knowledge is tested to demonstrate that the specialized knowledge and skills have been mastered.

Carcinogenicity studies Research that evaluates the potential of chemicals to induce carcinogenic (cancer causing) changes in rats and mice.

Caregiver An adult who provides care to someone who cannot take care of himself/herself; this can take the form of emotional or physical support.

Case report form (CRF) A document in which the results from a clinical trial are written (documented); the form may be paper or electronic. Data from the CRFs are analyzed at the end of the study.

Causality assessment The process by which the cause of an adverse event or serious adverse event is determined. Causality assessment involves assigning a probability or likelihood that the event or result was caused by the drug under study.

Cell The building block of the human body. Each cell contains organelles that are mini-factories which produce the materials needed by the body in order to function.

Cell membrane A critical part of the cell that forms a wall around it, controlling the substances that enter and leave the cell.

Chemical substance A material with a specific composition produced by a chemical process.

Chemotherapy The use of chemicals to treat disease.

Chromosome A long strand of DNA on which genes are found. Each human cell has 46 chromosomes in 23 pairs. One member of each pair is inherited from the mother, and the other is inherited from the father.

Chronic toxicity Side effects and adverse effects that occur after repeated administration of a pharmacologic agent.

Chronic toxicology studies Evaluations that involve the repeated administration of chemicals to animals to determine the toxicity profile.

Clinical endpoint Outcomes that are studied and documented during a clinical trial.

Clinical hold The formal cessation of a clinical trial by the Food and Drug Administration or prevention of a clinical trial from starting, usually due to safety concerns. The clinical hold can only be removed after the safety concerns have been addressed to the Food and Drug Administration's satisfaction.

Clinical investigation A systematic study of a drug designed to evaluate its safety and effectiveness (efficacy).

Clinical investigative site The hospital, doctor's office, or clinic where a clinical trial takes place.

Clinical investigator. *See also* **Sub-investigator** The physician who has the responsibility for the patient's well-being during a clinical trial. The clinical investigator must ensure that the clinical protocol is complied with and that the rights of research subjects are protected.

Clinical phases (1, 2, 3, 4) Clinical research is divided into four phases. Phase 1 often involves the administration of relatively small amounts of a drug to research subjects to determine how it works (pharmacology), its appropriate dose, and its pharmacokinetic profile. Phase 2 involves trying to determine an appropriate dose that will be safe and effective. Phase 3 studies involve the administration of the drug at the doses studied in Phase 2 to confirm efficacy and safety. Phase 4 studies are carried out after a therapeutic is marketed. These studies help to determine how the drug works in real life in a wider population than could be studied during clinical trials.

Clinical protocol A written "road map" that provides instructions to all involved with the conduct of the clinical trial on how it should be run.

Clinical protocol amendment A written description of changes to the clinical protocol that alters an aspect of how the clinical trial will be conducted.

Clinical research The process of studying a drug in research subjects.

Clinical research organization; Contract research organization (CRO) A service company hired by the sponsor to perform and oversee the clinical research on the sponsor's behalf and under the sponsor's supervision.

Clinical site; Investigative site This is the location (clinic, physician's office, or hospital) where a clinical trial takes place.

Clinical trial; Clinical study Research carried out in human subjects to determine if a drug is safe and/or effective.

Clinical trial application (CTA) A compilation of documentation submitted to health authorities in order to obtain permission to carry out a clinical trial in healthy volunteers and/or patients.

Clinical trial monitoring. *See also* **Monitoring** The process of oversight required by good clinical practice that calls for a clinical professional, who represents the sponsor, to visit the investigative site regularly and to monitor the results of the clinical study on an ongoing basis. Clinical trial monitoring involves making sure that the clinical protocol is being followed and that the rights of the research subjects are being protected.

Clinical trial study report A written description of the findings from a clinical trial.

Cognition The processes involved in thinking. The psychological ability to develop concepts.

Comparator A marketed medicine or placebo against which the drug under study is compared for safety and efficacy.

Compassionate use The provision of drugs to patients outside of a clinical trial, and before they are approved for marketing, for special cases.

Compliance The extent to which the trial procedures are followed. This term can also be applied in relation to the extent to which research subjects follow the study procedures and/or the instructions given for taking the drug.

Confidentiality Prevention of disclosure to other than authorized individuals of information that is private to the individual or sponsor.

Conflict of interest. *See also* **Financial conflict of interest; Financial interest** A situation in which a person responsible for conducting the clinical trial also has a financial interest in the outcome or results of the study.

Consent. *See also* **Informed consent form; Informed consent process** The act of agreeing to take part in a clinical trial or to undergo a procedure. To grant consent, individuals must have an understanding of the facts presented in the document that they will be required to sign, and they must have the mental capacity to understand the information presented.

Contract toxicology organization A service company that conducts toxicology studies on behalf of sponsors.

Contraindication A specific circumstance when the use of a certain treatment is to be avoided because of the relatively high likelihood of harm resulting.

Control group The group of research subjects in a randomized clinical trial who receive the standard treatment (the treatment that is already on the market) or a placebo. The observations for the drug under study will be compared with those from the control group.

Copyright A form of intellectual property that grants the originator the rights to distribute, market, and commercialize the copyrighted item for a specific period of time.

Corticosteroid (steroid) A medicine used to treat diseases that have an immunological component.

Cytosine One of the four bases in DNA, abbreviated as C. Cytosine always pairs with guanine. *See also* Base pairs.

Data exclusivity A period of time guaranteed to the originator of a new chemical entity, during which competitors cannot refer to or use the data that were compiled and filed to health authorities for approval.

Debilitate; Debilitating The act of making weak or feeble.

Dechallenge The act of stopping administration of a drug that is suspected to have caused an adverse event or serious adverse event.

Declaration of Helsinki A set of principles by which clinical research is conducted to ensure the ethical conduct of clinical research and the protection of research subjects.

Definitely related A causality assignment given when there is conclusive evidence that an adverse event or a serious adverse event was caused by the drug. In order for a definite causality to be assigned, the adverse event must resolve itself when the drug is removed or administration is stopped; the adverse event or serious adverse event must return when the drug is readministered.

Deoxyribonucleic acid (DNA) The nucleic acids that contain instructions that govern the functioning and development of living organisms.

Device; Medical device An instrument or material used to diagnose or treat a disease.

Diagnostic agent; Diagnostic test A drug or instrument used to identify disease and/or monitor it.

Documentation During drug development, results of the various studies conducted that are collated in electronic, hard copy (paper), X-rays, electro-cardiograms, optical, and other formats.

Dose–limiting toxicity (DLT) In some clinical trial designs, the drug is administered to research subjects at increasing doses until side effects and adverse events are severe enough that further increases in doses cannot be administered. The toxicity (adverse events/side effects) that results under these circumstances is known as dose-limiting toxicity.

Dose–ranging study A clinical trial in which two or more doses of a drug are studied. The purpose of a dose-range study is to determine the most appropriate dose to take forward into further clinical trials.

Double blind A design of a clinical trial in which neither the investigator nor the research subject knows which type of treatment is being received by the research subject.

Drug A pharmaceutical product that is being evaluated for safety and efficacy. The term *drug* used in this book is a catchall that includes medicinal products, devices, diagnostics, gene therapies, etc.

Drug development The process of developing a drug to determine if it is safe and effective enough to be commercialized for use in humans.

Drug discovery The process by which new chemical entities (new medicines) are found for the treatment of specific diseases.

Drug–drug interactions A situation in which one medicine affects the activity of another medicine by increasing or decreasing its activity, or increasing the activity of both drugs. Drug–drug interactions can cause adverse events and can be life threatening.

Drug registration. *See also* **Registration** The process of collating results gathered during the drug development process and submitting these documentation to the various health authorities in the countries where the sponsor intends to market the drug. This process involves the assessment and approval of the documentation, leading to the authorization for the drug to be marketed. if the necessary standard has been achieved

Efficacy Another term for effectiveness. It is used to describe the beneficial effect of a drug on a disease. Phase 2 studies are generally used to study efficacy effects. Phase 3 studies are used to confirm efficacy.

Elderly For purposes of clinical trial conduct, a person is considered elderly at 65 years of age.

Electrocardiograph (ECG) A device used to monitor the heart. It is used to identify diseases of the heart, the impact of drugs used to treat the heart, and the potential adverse effects of drugs on the heart.

Embryonic stem cells Cells that are obtained from aborted fetuses or fertilized eggs left over from in vitro fertilization. They can differentiate into different types of cells in the body.

Endpoint. *See also* **Clinical endpoint** A target outcome. For instance, for a blood pressure medicine, the reduction of blood pressure could be set as an important endpoint.

Enrollment. *See also* **Accrual** The process of including research subjects in a clinical trial. Before enrollment, research subjects are evaluated against the protocol's inclusion and exclusion criteria to determine if they can be enrolled in the clinical trial.

Ethics committee (EC) A group of experts that approves the protocol before the clinical trial can start. This group of experts oversees the clinical trial while it is ongoing to assure the safety of the research subjects in the clinical trial and to ensure that their ethical rights are protected.

Eukaryotic Cells that contain a nucleus.

European Medicines Evaluation Agency (EMEA/EMA) The regulatory authority that oversees the regulation of medicines in the European Union.

European Union (EU) An economic and political union of currently 27 countries in Europe.

Exceptional circumstances A category of regulatory approval in Europe that allows drugs which meet certain special criteria to be approved more quickly than under normal circumstances.

Exclusion criteria A set of conditions that if present in research subjects will lead them to be disqualified from taking part in a clinical trial.

Experimental drug A drug unproven in terms of its potential to produce a beneficial effect. This can also apply to the unproven nature of the drug in terms of its safety.

Experimental group The research subjects in a clinical trial who receive the drug being studied in a randomized clinical trial.

Family doctor. *See also* **General practitioner; Primary care physician** A physician who is trained to provide primary medical care.

Financial conflict of interest Situations in which monetary considerations may compromise or have the appearance of compromising a clinical investigator's clinical judgment.

Financial interest A situation in which a person has a financial stake in a sponsor or a program that is being developed. This can lead to a financial conflict of interest.

Food and Drug Administration (FDA) The U.S. government agency that enforces the Food, Drug and Cosmetics Act and related U.S. federal and public health laws. The FDA also grants approvals for investigational and New Drug applications.

Formulation The process by which a medicine is produced from the active ingredient. It can also refer to the pharmaceutical product administered to a research subject.

Gene A unit of inheritance. Together the genes make up the genome of an individual.

Gene expression This is the process by which protein and other molecules are produced from genes.

Gene therapy. *See also* **Gene transfer** An experimental therapy that involves the administration of genes into the human body to promote the production of proteins that may be missing or that may not be produced naturally in sufficient amounts.

Gene transfer The process of transferring genes into the human body for a therapeutic purpose.

General clinical research centers (GCRCs) A national network of centers (in the United States) within hospitals and research centers. They provide a research infrastructure for clinical investigators.

General practitioner (GP). *See also* **Family doctor** A physician trained to provide primary medical care.

Genetic code The set of rules encoded in genetic material that is translated into proteins and other material needed in order for the body to function appropriately.

Geriatrics The study of diseases that primarily affect the elderly, those who are over 65 years of age. This term is also used to refer to the discipline of physicians and health professionals involved with overseeing the medical care of the elderly.

Good clinical practice (GCP) All clinical trials must be conducted to a set of standards. These standards assure the protection of the human rights of research subjects. These standards provide guidance for the professionals involved with the oversight and conduct of clinical trials, and they assure the quality and accuracy of the data collected.

Good laboratory practice (GLP) This is a standard of conduct and documentation applied to animal toxicology, pharmacology and laboratory studies to assure the quality and accuracy of the data collected.

Good manufacturing practice (GMP) This is a standard applied to the manufacture of drugs intended for humans. It involves assuring that material to be administered to research subjects and patients is manufactured to an appropriately high standard. This standard also includes ensuring that all aspects of the manufacturing process are documented in detail.

Guanine One of the four bases in DNA, abbreviated as G. Guanine always pairs with cytosine. *See also* Base pairs.

Guideline; Guidance; Notice to Applicants; Points to consider Guidance provided to sponsors by regulatory authorities to provide information on best drug development practices.

Health authority. *See also* **Regulatory authority** Governmental agencies that have the responsibility for assuring the quality, safety, and efficacy of drugs for use in humans.

Health Insurance Portability and Accountability Act (HIPAA) Legislation passed in the United States in 1996 that includes a privacy rule creating national standards to protect personal health information.

Health status The state of health of an individual. This may be determined using physical examination, questionnaires, and other forms of tests.

Healthy volunteer/Normal volunteer A research subject who has a good health status. In clinical trials they help to determine how the drug acts on a human body without the disease under study.

Hypoglycemic The state of having a lower blood sugar level than one should have. This occurs in diabetics when the administration of insulin or antidiabetic drugs may reduce blood sugar to too low a level.

Imaging The visual representation of a body part for the purposes of medical diagnosis or treatment of a disease. Some examples of techniques that can be used for imaging purposes are computerized tomography (CT) scans, X-rays, sonography, and ultrasound.

Inclusion criteria A set of criteria against which research subjects are screened in order to determine if they are eligible for enrollment in a clinical trial.

Informed A state of being knowledgeable or educated about a subject or matter.

Informed consent document; Informed consent form A document signed by research subjects before they can participate in a clinical trial. It outlines the details of the study, potential risks, and any evidence for efficacy.

Informed consent process The process by which the principal investigator or staff explain the contents of the informed consent document to the research subject. It is the process by which research subjects voluntarily confirm willingness to participate in a particular clinical trial. Informed consent is documented by the research subject by signing and dating an informed consent form. The process of obtaining informed consent is ongoing during the clinical trial.

Inhaler A device used to deliver a drug to the lungs.

Inspection – A systemic review of data and documentation carried out by a health authority to determine if the data at the investigative sites or manufacturing facilities were collected correctly, and are consistent with the data in the application.

Institutional biosafety committee (IBC). *See also* **Biosafety committee** A committee that reviews the documentation for gene therapy and experimental approaches which are biological in nature to assure that the drug is safe enough to be handled by the health care professionals at the investigative site and that it is safe enough to be administered to research subjects.

Institutional review board (IRB). *See also* **Ethics committee** In most countries this committee is known as an ethics committee. An independent group of medical and scientific experts as well as lay members who review and approve clinical protocols before clinical trials can start. This group of experts oversees the clinical trial while it is ongoing to assure the safety of the research subjects in the clinical trial and to ensure that their ethical rights are protected.

Investigational new drug (IND) application An application consisting of the information that is known about a drug, including in vitro and animal studies at the time of submission. This documentation is submitted by a sponsor to the Food and Drug Administration in order to obtain permission to carry out a clinical trial in research subjects (healthy volunteers and/or patients).

Investigative site; Investigational site. *See also* **Clinical site** The location (clinic, physician's office, or hospital) where a clinical trial takes place.

Investigator. *See also* **Clinical investigator; Principal investigator (PI)** The physician who has the responsibility for the patient's well-being during a clinical trial. The clinical investigator must ensure that the clinical protocol is complied with and that the rights of the research subject are protected.

Investigator's brochure The document that provides professionals involved with running the clinical trial with the scientific background required to ensure the safe and effective conduct of the clinical trial.

Juvenile toxicology studies Evaluations conducted in very young animals to the standards of good laboratory practice to determine how the drug might affect pediatric patients administered to them

Licensing agreement A legally binding contract that details the terms by which a drug or medicine is licensed out by one party to another for drug development.

Life threatening A disease or condition that puts a person's life at risk of ending prematurely.

Magnetic resonance imaging machine (MRI) A diagnostic scanning technique that produces detailed images of internal tissues by analyzing its response to being bombarded with high-frequency radio waves within a strong magnetic field.

Marketing authorization application (MAA). *See also* **New drug application (NDA)** An application that is submitted after all studies in animals and humans are completed. The regulatory authorities review the application and provide an approval for marketing (commercialization) if the data indicate that the drug is safe, effective, and manufactured to a good quality.

Medical history A detailed review of a patient's medical past, including any illnesses, surgeries, and medications taken.

Medication history A detailed review of the medicines taken to treat illnesses in the medical history.

Medicine In this book, the term used to indicate a commercially available drug that has successfully completed all necessary testing in animals and humans, and that has proven to be safe, efficacious, and of a good quality by regulatory authorities.

Membrane A thin layer that is present outside organelles within the cell and also outside large organs in the body.

Messenger RNA A molecule in the cell that transports the information to the ribosomes, where protein is produced, telling them which protein to make.

Metabolism. *See also* **ADME** The chemical reactions that occur in cells to break down chemicals that are ingested by human beings and animals.

Ministry of Health and Welfare (MHW) The regulatory authority that oversees the regulation of medicines in Japan.

Molecular biology The study of biology on a molecular level.

Monitoring The act of overseeing the clinical trial to ensure it is conducted in accordance with good clinical practice (GCP).

Monoamine oxidase inhibitor (MAOI) A class of medicines used to treat severe depression by correcting chemical imbalances.

Multicenter; Multicentre Involving several investigative sites at the same time. The same clinical protocol will be followed at each investigative site.

Multinational Involving several different countries at the same time. The same clinical protocol will be followed in each country and at each investigative site.

Mutagenicity studies Research carried out to determine if a chemical or drug is able to damage DNA.

National Institutes of Health (NIH) U.S. Government–funded agency that conducts biomedical and health-related research.

National Institute of Mental Health (NIMH) U.S. Government–funded agency focused on research in the area of mental health.

New chemical entity (NCE) A drug that contains an active component that has not been registered (approved) by the regulatory authority; it is therefore considered a new chemical entity.

New drug application (NDA). *See also* **Marketing authorization application (MAA)** An application submitted after all studies in animals and humans are completed. The Food and Drug Administration and other health authorities review the documentation and provide an approval for marketing (commercialization) if the data indicate that the drug is safe and effective.

Normal volunteers. *See also* **Healthy volunteers** Research subjects who have good health status. They help to determine how the drug acts on the human body without the presence of the disease for which the drug under study is being developed.

Not related A causality assignment given when there is conclusive evidence that an adverse event or a serious adverse event was not caused by the drug. In order for a not-related causality to be assigned, there must be other plausible causes for the adverse event besides the drug.

Nucleolus A non-membrane-bound part of the cell nucleus.

Nucleus The control center of the cell.

Off-label use When a product is used in a way or to treat a disease that has not been authorized by a regulatory authority.

Open-label trial A trial that is not blinded. Both the investigators and the patients know which treatment is being administered to the research subject. An open-label clinical trial may be randomized or non-randomized.

Operons A group of key nucleotide sequences including an operator, a common promoter, and one or more structural genes that are controlled as a unit to produce messenger RNA.

Organelles A special structure in a cell that has a function. Each organelle is enclosed within its own membrane.

Orphan disease A disease that occurs rarely.

Over the counter (OTC) Medicines that are available without a prescription but that are sold under the supervision of pharmacists.

Oversight The process of providing supervision.

Patent A set of rights granted to an inventor for a limited period of time in exchange for a disclosure of an invention.

Patient A research subject who has the disease under study.

Patient advocate A person who liaises between the patient and the physician and other health care providers to ensure the needs of the patient or research subject are met.

Pharmaceutical Relates to the manufacture, study, and use of medicines to treat disease.

Pharmacokinetics (PK) The process that the body uses to absorb, excrete, metabolize, and distribute the drug within the body.

Pharmacology The study of the activity of drugs.

Phase 1 (Phase I) clinical trial The initial studies conducted to determine the metabolism and pharmacologic actions of drugs. These studies may include healthy volunteers or patients.

Phase 2 (Phase II) clinical trial The studies carried out to determine the efficacy of drugs. These studies are carried out in patients with the disease or condition under study.

Phase 3 (Phase III) clinical trial The larger confirmatory studies carried out in patients with the disease under study to confirm efficacy. They are usually controlled.

Phase 4 (Phase IV) clinical trial The postmarketing studies to determine additional benefits for the drug.

Physician A medically qualified individual.

Placebo A preparation that is pharmacologically inert or lacking in an active pharmaceutical ingredient. A placebo has no treatment value.

Placebo effect A beneficial effect that occurs in a disease state or disorder after a placebo is administered instead of a drug.

Possibly related A causality assignment given when there is a temporal and plausible link between an adverse event or a serious adverse event and a drug.

Preclinical Referring to processes, research, and testing of experimental drugs in animals before testing in humans.

Prevalence The total number of cases of the disease in the population at a given time, or the total number of cases in the population, divided by the number of individuals in the population.

Primary care physician. *See also* **Family doctor; General practitioner** A doctor trained to provide primary medical care.

Principal investigator (PI) The physician responsible for the oversight of a clinical trial at an investigative site and sometimes at a number of investigative sites. The principal investigator must ensure that the clinical protocol is complied with and that the rights of the research subjects are protected. The principal investigator oversees the sub-investigators.

Privacy Steps taken to ensure that medical information belonging to one person is protected from transmission to others who have no appropriate reason to see it.

Probably related A causality assignment given when there is a temporal and plausible link between an adverse event or a serious adverse event and a drug. A removal of the drug (dechallenge) will lead to resolution of the adverse event or serious adverse event. For safety reasons, it may not be feasible to risk readministering the drug to see if a definite causality assignment is appropriate.

Prokaryotes A group of organisms that lack a nucleus (e.g., bacteria).

Protocol. *See also* **Clinical protocol** A written "road map" that provides instructions to all involved with the conduct of the clinical trial on how it should be run.

Quackery Unproven or fraudulent claims.

Quality assurance (QA) The process of ensuring that the toxicology studies, clinical trials, and manufacturing are conducted to good laboratory practice, good clinical practice standards, good manufacturing practice, and that other regulatory requirements are complied with.

Quality of life An area of clinical research that involves the determination of the effect of a drug on the quality of a person's life.

Randomization The process by which the research subject is assigned to receive either the drug containing the pharmaceutical ingredient or placebo. This is carried out by a process involving chance to reduce bias.

Randomized clinical trial A clinical trial in which research subjects are assigned by chance to the group in which the drug is administered or the group in which the placebo or comparator is administered.

Rare disease A disease that occurs at a frequency which is considered rare.

Registration. *See also* **Drug registration** The process of collating the results gathered during the drug development process and submitting this documentation to the various health authorities in the countries in which the sponsor intends to market the drug. This process involves the assessment and approval of the documentation, providing the authorization for the drug to be marketed.

Regulations Rules issued by governments to oversee the research and development of drugs.

Regulatory authority. *See also* **Health authorities** Governmental agencies that have the responsibility for assuring the quality, safety, and efficacy of medicines and drugs intended for use in humans.

Reproductive toxicology The study of the effects of chemicals on the reproductive and neuroendocrine systems, as well as the embryo, fetus, neonate, and prepubertal animal that is being studied.

Research subject An individual who participates in a clinical trial. This person may be a healthy volunteer or a patient.

Ribosomes A small structure present within cells that is involved with the production of proteins.

Risk–benefit ratio A calculation that weighs a drug's negative (risk) and positive (benefit) effects depending on the disease, the medicine, and the health of the subject.

Rough endoplasmic reticulum (RER) An organelle within the cell involved with the production of proteins.

Serious adverse drug reaction A noxious and unintended response to a drug that occurs at any dose and requires inpatient hospitalization or prolongation of existing hospitalization, causes congenital malformation, results in persistent or significant disability or incapacity, is life-threatening, or results in death.

Serious adverse event (SAE) An untoward medical occurrence that at any dose results in death, is life-threatening, requires inpatient hospitalization or prolongs existing hospitalization, results in persistent or significant disability/incapacity, or causes a congenital abnormality.

Side effect An undesired effect that occurs from a medicine or drug as a result of its pharmacological action.

Single blind A design of a clinical trial in which the investigator is aware of the treatment that is being administered to each research subject. The research subjects do not know which treatments they are receiving.

Site management organization (SMO) An organization that oversees the investigative site to ensure that it meets appropriate standards of good clinical practice.

Source data Original medical records and certified copies of original medical records.

Species–specific effects Effects that occur uniquely in one species but not in others.

Sponsor An individual, company, institution, or organization responsible for the initiation, management, and financing of a clinical trial.

Standard operating procedures Detailed written processes for the conduct of various aspects of drug development that ensure that everyone involved with the clinical trial follows a standard or uniform set of procedures.

Stopping rules Guidelines built into the clinical protocol that explain the circumstances under which a clinical trial will be stopped to assure the safety of the research subjects.

Sub-acute toxicology; Sub-chronic toxicology The study of noxious (toxic) findings after the repeated administration of a drug for limited periods of time.

Sub-investigator. *See also* **Clinical investigator; Principal investigator** A physician who is part of the clinical trial team. This physician works under the supervision of the principal investigator as far as the clinical trial is concerned. The sub-investigator must ensure that the clinical protocol is complied with and that the rights of the research subject are protected.

Target organ The organ that is most adversely affected by the drug during animal toxicology studies.

Terminal cancer A form of cancer that cannot be cured by treatment, although it may be possible to treat its symptoms.

Terminally ill A patient who is suffering from an incurable disease.

Therapeutic; Therapeutic agent A drug used to treat, diagnose, or cure disease. In this book, the term *drug* includes medicines, devices, diagnostics, and other therapeutic modalities.

Thymine One of the four bases in DNA, abbreviated to T. Thymine always pairs with adenine. *See also* Base pairs.

Toxicity An adverse effect of a drug.

Toxicology The study of the adverse effects of chemicals on animals and living organisms. It usually involves the administration of higher doses to the animals and organisms than will normally be administered to human beings to determine their adverse effects and potential side effects.

Trademark A distinctive mark used to brand a product.

Transplantation The removal of an organ from one human being in order to place it in another. This is usually accompanied by the administration of immunosuppressant drugs to prevent organ rejection.

Trial site. *See also* **Clinical site; Investigative site, Investigational site** The hospital, clinic, or physician's office where the clinical trial is conducted.

Unexpected adverse drug effect or reaction An unforeseen and undesirable effect or reaction that occurs after a drug is administered; it has not been observed before and is therefore not documented in the investigator's brochure for drugs that are not marketed or the product label/summary of product characteristics for marketed products.

Unmet medical needs Usually a serious illness or disease for which there is no current treatment or for which current treatment is inadequate in terms of curing the disease or controlling symptoms of the disease.

Venture capital firms (VCs) Companies that provide funds to sponsor companies to underwrite the research and development of drugs. They are active investors in pharmaceutical and biotechnological research, especially for smaller companies. They select their investments in a discerning way to increase the chances of making a profit if the research and development is successful.

Vital signs Important measurements taken during a clinical trial to measure the impact of a drug on the research subject's body. They include blood pressure, heart rate, temperature, etc.

Xenotransplantation Transplantation of organs from an animal source into the human body. This area of research must be considered experimental.

Index

Note: Page numbers followed by "*f*" and "*t*" denote figures and tables, respectively.